傷寒論序

傷寒論。蓋祖述大聖人之意。諸家莫其倫擬。故晉皇甫謐序甲乙鍼經云。伊尹以元聖之才。撰用神農本草。以為湯液。漢張仲景論廣湯液。為十數卷。用之多驗。近世太醫令王叔和。撰次仲景遺論甚精。皆可施用。是仲景本伊尹之法。伊尹本神農之經。得不謂祖述大聖人之意乎。張仲景漢書無傳。見名醫錄云。南陽人。名機。仲景乃其字也。舉孝廉。官至長沙太守。始受術於同郡張伯祖。時人言。識用精微過其師。所著論。其言精而奧。其法簡而

KAMPO

How the Japanese Updated
Traditional Herbal Medicine

Akira Tsumura

KAMPO

How the Japanese Updated Traditional Herbal Medicine

漢方

Japan Publications, Inc.

Note to the reader Those with health problems are advised to seek the guidance of a qualified medical or psychological professional before implementing any of the approaches presented in this book. It is essential that any readers, who have any reason to suspect serious illness in themselves or their family members seek appropriate medical, nutritional, or psychological advice promptly. Neither this or any other health related book should be used as a substitute for qualified care or treatment.

Editorial Direction: Albert H. Matano
Editors: Caroline Crane, Russell Palmer, Barbara L. Jurin-Reid
Botanical Drawings by Frank Fretz, from Rodales's *Illustrated Encyclopedia of Herbs*
Photographs of Herbs and Minerals from Tsumura's *Kampo Handbook*

Productive Direction: Random Inc.

Published by Japan Publications, Inc., Tokyo and New York

Distributors:
UNITED STATES: Kodansha America, Inc. through Farrar, Straus & Giroux, 19 Union Square West, New York 10003. CANADA: Fitzhenry & Whiteside Ltd., 195 Allstate Parkway, Markham, Ontario, L3R 4T8. BRITISH ISLES AND EUROPEAN CONTINENT: Premier Book Marketing Ltd., 1 Gower Street, London WC1E 6HA. AUSTRALIA AND NEW ZEALAND: Bookwise International, 54 Crittenden Road, Findon, South Australia 5023. THE FAR EAST AND JAPAN: Japan Publications Trading Co., Ltd., 1-2-1, Sarugaku-cho, Chiyoda-ku, Tokyo 101.

First Edition: September 1991
ISBN 0-87040-792-9
LCCC 91-060181

Printed in Japan

TABLE OF CONTENTS

Preface

Modern medicine is in crisis. Many factors, including a shortage of qualified nurses and the shocking escalation of costs, have lessened the chances that the average citizen of the U.S. can be sure of getting proper hospital care.

What can be done? The public is seeking the answer in health food stores, exercise studios, and in new fields of medicine.

There is a growing interest in good, old-fashioned herbal remedies. Herbs have been used safely for centuries throughout the world, primarily as part of a program of preventive medicine, reducing the cost of treatment all along the line. Oddly, herbs work best in cases that baffle medical science, from mental illness to the common cold. They work a kinder, gentler cure, making them especially well suited for the treatment of our growing numbers of senior citizens.

The truth is that although western medicine is good at managing trauma, acute bacterial infections, surgical emergencies and other crises, it is tragically limited in its ability to manage viral infections, chronic degenerative diseases, allergies, cancer, and mental illness.

For these and many more reasons the World Health Organization (WHO) is urging member governments to develop a "New Medicine" combining the ancient arts of the herbalist with modern science. The idea has proven merit. In Japan, the old and the new medicine have been bedfellows since 1976 with spectacular results. In fact, Kampo medications have become a widely accepted means of healing even in our hi-tech society.

In our scientific laboratories, researchers using the latest technology are busy analyzing the properties of popular Kampo remedies to find the key to their success and are constantly upgrading their production. Age-old Kampo remedies are now processed in the most modern, hi-tech facilities. Additional research on herbal remedies has begun on a large scale in China, West Germany, and in the Third World as well. To most of the English-speaking world, however, Kampo remains an Oriental mystery.

Those who wish to explore that mystery can find a basic guide to the Japanese experience with medicinal herbs in these pages.

Introduction

There's no doubt in my mind that nature's herbs will revolutionize modern medicine within a surprisingly short time. Already new herbal drugs show promise in the war on cancer, and aids.

That is why we worked hard to make this book on the Japanese art of herbal healing as complete and helpful as possible. You'll find the most important aspects of this ancient discipline discussed along with its promise for the future. All simplified for the layman.

In Parts I and II you'll learn from our Japanese experience how traditional herbalism and modern western medicine can co-exist, to the benefit of both. You'll learn why the medical profession and the public worldwide are now exploring the whole field of healing with herbal medicine with unprecedented fervor.

Why such enthusiasm? Herbs are helping researchers find new cures every day for a host of illnesses. In addition, we've included some actual case histories of Westerners who have been treated by Kampo physicians and have found it a welcome change from western medicine's usual impersonal drug therapy.

Strange as it seems, western medicine is least successful in dealing with the ills of modern man brought on by stress, faulty diet, and longer life. Here, nature's own healing herbs do best. In Part III you'll find an analysis of eighteen common contemporary illnesses, and a summary of how they respond to western medicine's drugs and to the more gentle Kampo medications. How do they compare? There are a lot of surprises in these pages for the reader!

For the serious student of herbal healing, Part IV offers the names, basic pharmaceutical content, and uses of traditional unrefined herbal cures, and also the modern refined herbal mixtures found equally effective by today's Kampo physicians.

Listings in the back will help those who wish to explore further on their own.

One caution: Our intent in this book is to give background information, not to diagnose or prescribe. We suggest you get professional medical care if you have a serious illness or are menopausal, pregnant, or think you may be pregnant. Do not attempt to take herbal cures if you are already under medication without consulting a doctor.

AKIRA TSUMURA

"There is an herb for every illness."

—Abbé Sebastian Kneipp

Why Herbal Medicine? A History

Herbs have been used to cure illness since the dawn of man.

In primitive societies, shamans still know and use plants that heal in the green pharmacy that is their home. On a recent expedition to Brazil, to learn more about healing herbs before the great Amazon rain forest is destroyed, U.S. scientists from the Smithsonian Institution were shown new cures for ear ache, diarrhea, and eye disorders. Chances are, hidden deep in the jungle, are cures for almost every disease known to man. (At this moment a Chinese herb holding promise of curing AIDS is being tested in modern laboratories.)

The first written reference to herbs is the story of a Chinese farmer who seriously wounded a large snake that threatened his farm animals. The next day, the snake was back again, completely rejuvenated. When the farmer "fatally wounded" the snake again, he was amazed to find it returning the next day. He watched from a hiding place and discovered the snake's secret. He saw the wounded, bleeding snake crawl into a bed of weeds, eat the leaves, and slowly regain its strength. To this day, Chinese soldiers carry these same leaves into battle to help them recover from the wounds of war. They call the plant *Jin bu huan*, or "gold-no-trade."

The early Egyptians, Romans, and Greeks all knew the value of herbal medicine. Hippocrates, Galen, and Pliny the Elder all included herbal remedies in their writings. In India, herbal medicine is vital to the ancient healing art of Ayurveda.

The Aztec's herb book, written in pictograms, was destroyed by the Spanish conquistadores. A similar fate wiped out the record of herbal cures in Wales when the British invaded and tried to destroy the Welsh culture. In Imperial Rome, the gladiators drank fennel tea to build strength—safely—centuries before steroids.

In North America, early explorers traded know-how with the native American Indians. The tribes taught them which herbs to use to sharpen their senses for hunting, to build endurance, and to bait their traps. The Jesuits dug up the plentiful American ginseng, sold it to the Chinese, and used the money to build schools and churches.

Today, in Pakistan, traditional medicine known as Unani Tibb is accepted as a state system alongside modern western medical treatments. In Vietnam, families are being encouraged to grow "family medicine" plants in each village. As a result of government studies there to evaluate the true healing properties of native plants, forty new remedies for such diverse ailments as high blood pressure, rheumatism, hepatitis, goiter, coughs, allergy, and shock have been pioneered in the last decade. Bangladesh, Madagascar, Rwanda, Thailand, and other Third World countries are starting similar programs. In Africa, 95% of traditional drugs come from plants.

The Chinese made the first great leap forward in herbal medicine. They explored the use of thousands of herbs and made the first written record covering the use of herbs for healing, the *Pen T'sao Ching* (Materia Medica), by the legendary Emperor Shen Nang, circa 3000 B.C.

The early Chinese were the first to discover that plants did not always use one active ingredient to heal but often depended on the action and interaction of dozens of chemical ingredients. (This was the origin of Chinese polypharmacy.) For example, the Ghanian *Cryptolepis sanguinolenta* reduces fever, cures urinary infections, and acts as a broad spectrum antibiotic—yet none of the individual substances isolated from it is a recognizable antibiotic. It is the combination of ingredients that is so effective. This, of course, runs contrary to western thought which prefers one problem, one cure.

Significantly, the Chinese shifted the emphasis of treatment to the prevention of illness. Just eradicating the symptoms of disease is not enough. The patient must be restored to a healthy life through harmony with nature. This is their idea of Tao. (Westerners might use the term "holism".)

The Chinese also became masters of diagnosis through palpation, or exploration of the patient's body by touch. Through palpation by a highly trained diagnostician, the state of the deep, inner organs of the body can be discerned. The hands of the practitioner become highly sensitized through long, vigorous training. Skin qualities, muscle shapes, tendons, blood vessels, and anastomoses, lymph vessels and nodes are among the multitude of clues Asian physicians receive through palpation.

In Japan, this rich heritage of thousands of years in the prevention of disease was adopted as Kampo medicine and made a part of our culture. Simply stated, the art of Kampo healing is based on the principle that the human organism possesses the inherent ability to protect, regulate, and heal itself. This innate wisdom is the vital life force (*vis medicatrix naturae*). During a consultation, the herbalist seeks to indentify in which respect this vital force has been breached.

Such an assessment today makes use of diagnostic techniques, equipment, and clinical tests common to orthodox medicine plus a careful questioning about the patient's past history, diet, and lifestyle. It is remarkably complete and valid for further treatment.

The gentle, harmonizing effect of herbal medicines, which provide necessary trace elements, vitamins, and medicinal substances, then starts the rehabilitation process. Kampo treatment differs from the usual orthodox medical care in other ways: The Kampo physician interprets symptoms as a manifestation of the efforts of the vital life force to return the body to health and so seeks to aid this process rather than simply suppress them.

Japan is now a leader in the field of "New Medicine," blending the best of western and Asian schools. Gradually, it has eliminated traces of folk superstition associated with Chinese medicine. Japan is also a leader in researching the medicinal properties of tropical plants. There are three active research centers devoted exclusively to medicinal herbs in our country today. As far back as 1937, the isolation of *diosgenin* from the yam, *Dioscorea tokoro*, by Japanese researchers provided the basis of the modern contraceptive pill industry. Kampo and modern medical science make strange bedfellows, but they do coexist in Japan. And it is inevitable that they will in the United States and Europe as well. When that time comes, those who suffer needlessly from debilitating illnesses and from the effects of synthetic drugs that do violence to us as they heal can look for relief at last.

PART ONE

What is Kampo?

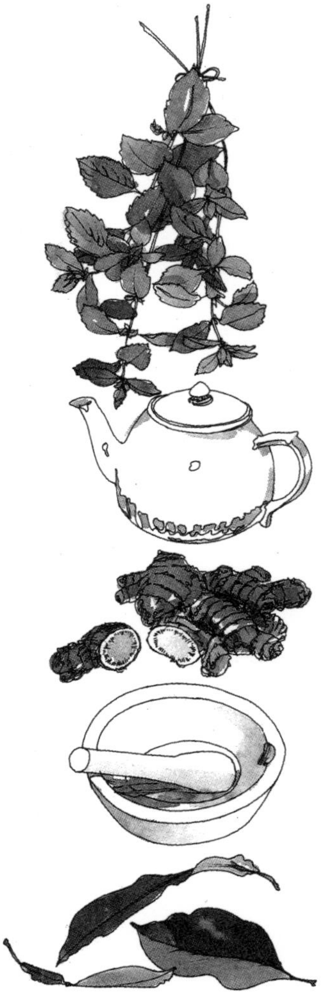

NOTE: *The transliteration of words from any language is not easy, nor uniform. Kampo is composed of two Chinese characters transliterated (or romanized based on the Hepburn system) into two unaccented syllables: kan and po as found in Japanese-English dictionaries. Combined they are pronounced kam po. The Japanese choose to transliterate it kampo and that is the way it will look throughout this book.*

Also, the terms "allopathic medicine," "orthodox medicine," and "western medicine" in our text all refer to modern medicine as practiced in the western world, based to a large extent on the use of powerful drugs and surgery.

"O plants and herbs! You have the power to rescue the sufferer.
I call upon you to make the remedy I prepare powerful and effective."

—Atharva Veda

CHAPTER 1

THE JAPANESE FOUNTAIN OF YOUTH

According to recent research conducted by the World Health Organization (WHO), the Japanese people are among the longest-lived in the world. Japanese men are found to live an average of 76 years, and women an average of 81.

Why is this so? No one knows exactly. Among the many factors contributing to longevity are diet and health care. This is one reason why health-conscious Americans are taking an interest in food such as fish and rice, which are featured heavily in the Japanese diet, and in Oriental medical disciplines such as acupuncture and moxa treatments (moxibustion).

An important part of Asian medicine is Kampo, a system of healing with natural herbs which are combined into remedies for specific ailments and designed individually for each patient. Today there are 170,000 medical practitioners in Japan. Of these, in spite of their western medical training, approximately 42.7 percent, or 72,590, prescribe Kampo medicine. The number of doctors specializing in Kampo is increasing rapidly.

Many books and articles about Kampo are currently available in Japanese bookstores. The new popularity of Kampo has come about largely for the following reasons: 1) A number of Kampo medications have been approved by the Japanese government and the cost of these treatments is now covered under the National Health Insurance System; 2) Because of this insurance coverage, Kampo medicines are now more affordable; 3) As a result of research by various Japanese pharmaceutical companies, Kampo medications are now available in more easily handled forms such as capsules; 4) The use of Kampo not only helps to cure many chronic diseases still considered incurable in orthodox medical circles, such as those associated with aging, but can also counteract the side effects of many new drugs.

CHAPTER 2

THE HISTORY OF KAMPO

There were two types of medicine in ancient China; pharmacotherapy, or the use of medicines, and physiotherapy, which included treatments such as acupuncture and moxibustion, in which herbs are burned at specific acupuncture points. Both fields are a part of what we refer to today as "Asian medicine."

During the Han Dynasty (206 B.C.–220 A.D.), the use of Kampo in clinics became widespread and it was soon established as the medical treatment of the time. Written records of Kampo during this period appear in such books as *The Yellow Emperor's Manual of Corporeal Medicine* (*Huang Ti Nei Ching*) and *The Pharmacopoeia of Heavenly Husbandry* (*Shen Nung Pen Ts'ao*).

The *Yellow Emperor's Manual* is known to be the oldest Chinese medical text, although the author remains anonymous. It is divided into two parts: one, called *Sumen*, which deals with the causes and types of illness; the other, called *Ling Shu* which contains diagnostic procedures and explains the technical skills of acupuncture and moxibustion. The *Manual* also contains sections dealing with the treatment of psychological disorders and mental defects.

The *Pharmacopoeia* notes 365 varieties of medicine, one for each day of the year. It is the oldest known pharmacopoeia and is divided into three sections.

> *Joyaku*, or Upper Class Medicine, is considered the most important section. It includes 120 different remedies containing nourishment for a robust life. These medicines are said to increase longevity when taken regularly over a period of time. All are harmless, producing no side effects.
>
> *Chuyaku*, or Middle Class Medicine, contains 120 formulas that are said to regenerate energy and keep the body healthy. These medicines do sometimes produce side effects and must be used with caution.
>
> *Shimoyaku*, or Lower Class Medicine, contains 125 formulas. Because of the

side effects caused by these medications, treatment cannot be continued over a long period of time.

These sections are in accordance with ancient Chinese healing practices which categorized medicine into three types: robust, health-maintenance, and treatment. In Kampo, the three are unified in physical and mental diagnosis.

Zhang Zing-jing wrote two medical texts: *Shang Han Lun*, which contains treatments for acute fevers and illness, and *Jin Kui Yao Lue*, which describes treatments for chronic diseases. The prescriptions for these treatments were taken from the *Pharmacopoeia*.

During the T'ang Dynasty (618–907 A.D.), two more books were written, *Chien Chin Fang* and *Wai Tai Pi Yao Fang*, both of which contain the prescriptions and secret methods of the famous practitioners of the time. In *Wai Tai Pi Yao Fang* are explanations of such treatments as acupuncture, moxibustion, and massage points.

The Reformation of Chinese Medicine

The period of the Sung Dynasty (960–1279 A.D.) and the Chin and Yuan Dynasty (1115–1368 A.D.) saw the systemization of Chinese medical theories and the creation of various schools. During the first half of the Sung Dynasty, the theories of Yin and Yang and the "Five Elements" arose. Later both theories were joined together and renamed the "Yin/Yang Five Element Theory." This theory, which is unlike anything known to modern orthodox medical practice, became the main basis of Chinese medicine, and was applied to the diagnosis and treatment of most diseases.

Also during the Sung Dynasty, the learned Chen Shih Wen wrote a book which was used as a text for the prescription of drugs and the diagnosis and treatment of diseases.

During the Manchu Dynasty (1662–1911 A.D.), no medical texts were written. Instead, there was a revival of the old texts and a slight departure from pure clinical medicine to researching those old texts.

At the same time, Japanese medicine was being studied in China. The Chinese practitioners were very interested in the concept of Fukushin or examination of the abdomen by palpation which was practiced by Japanese doctors.

During the early part of the 20th century, under the influence of orthodox medicine, a new scientific systematization of Chinese medical practices was established. As a result, the influence of Chinese medicine in Japan began to decline.

The Era of Imitation: Kampo Medicine in Japan

The traditional medicine of ancient China was brought to Japan by way of Korea. The Empress Suiko, whose reign began in 593 A.D., sent armies to invade Korea, where Chinese medicine was already in use. So impressed were the Japanese by the new medical practices they found there that later in her reign the Empress sent two representatives to study medicine in China.

More and more information about Chinese medicine began to reach Japan. During the Nara Period (710–794 A.D.), a Japanese Buddhist priest returned from China where he had been studying and told of the medical treatments he had seen. Japanese envoys came back from their voyages to China with news of the healing practices there. Until this time, incantation and prayer had been the main form of medical treatment in Japan.

During the Heian Period (794–1192 A.D.), Yasunori Tamba revised the oldest Japanese medical text, *Isshinho* (The Way of Medicine), drawing upon Chinese texts such as Chien Chin Fang. The result was a work of thirty volumes.

Influence of Medicine from the Chin and Yuan Dynasty

During the period from 1200 to 1600 A.D., medicine in Japan became more positive and practical. Buddhist medicine was the major influence and monks and priests were the main practitioners.

In addition to men of religion, specialists such as Sanki Tashiro appeared in the medical field. These were the students of the envoys who had gone to China to study medicine. They had a tremendous influence on the further development of medicine in Japan. During this entire period, the field of medicine progressed very rapidly. The Japanese further developed the Chinese medicine they had learned from the Chin and Yuan Dynasty era in addition to creating their own healing methods and researching the best of orthodox medicine from Europe.

The Japanese Version of Chinese Medicine

Dosan Manase, a student of Sanki Tashiro, carried on the practices of his teacher and created a Japanese version of the clinical treatments that had their origins in Buddhism. Dosan wrote a text called *Shuhokiku*, which was used as a reference guide by numerous doctors. It included many Kampo herbal treatments (Bing Hui Chun.)

The medicine of the Tokugawa (Shogun) Period [1603–1867 A.D.] centered around two schools: Gosei-ha and Koho-ha. Dosan's school, the Gosei-ha, derived its name from the medical schools of China in the Chin and Yuan Dynasties.

The Koho-ha school, based upon the text of the old *Shang Han Lun*, had its main location in Kyoto. Among its leaders were Konzan Goto, Shuan Kagawa, Toyo Yamawaki, and Ikkansai Matsubara.

Konzan taught himself medicine and created his own philosophy, which can be summarized by the comment: "Diseases are created when even one sense fails." This is similar to the old saying, "Sickness comes from anxiety." Konzan believed that disease could be cured when the senses were able to function smoothly and freely. His treatments consisted of moxibustion and hot spring baths. This type of treatment, he maintained, should precede the use of medicine.

Konzan's first student was Toyo Yamawaki. Later, he was the first in Japan to perform an autopsy. Toyo recorded his work in a book entitled *Zoshin* (Internal Organs). Another student, Shuan Kagawa, combined the practices of Confucianism and medicine.

Todo Yoshimasu was another influential practitioner whose philosophy was: "Thousands of diseases, one toxin." He believed that a person became ill because of toxins, or poisons that entered the body. Once the body was able to rid itself of these poisons, it would be cured. This was accomplished by taking a counter-toxin, otherwise known as medicine. If toxins remained in the body, Todo believed, the symptoms would appear in the abdomen.

Thus, Japan had its own version of abdominal examination. Sometimes a form of poison was used to rid the body of toxins. Often a patient would lose consciousness as a result of the poison. This was called Meigen, or Dark Faint. It was said that after such a loss of consciousness, the patient would be cured.

Todo recorded this procedure in two works: *Yakubi* (Collection of Medicines), and *Ruishuho* (Varieties of Medicine). *Yakubi* describes the effects and benefits of Kampo, as listed in the *Shang Han Lun=Jin Kui Yao Lue*, and *Ruishuho* notes the applications of Kampo.

Orthodox Medicine and the Decline of Kampo

During the Meiji Period (1868–1912 A.D.), European culture began to work its way into Japan. Military affairs became the country's central concern bringing about the creation of military medicine. Kampo medicine, in which no surgery is performed, began to decline in popularity. In 1883, Kampo was virtually abandoned because physicians were required to have licenses in order to practice, and the government, which granted those licenses, was uninterested in nonsurgical medicine.

The Revival of Kampo Medicine

In 1910, a book called *Ikai No Tekken* (Fundamentals in the Medical Field), by Keijuro Wada, spoke very highly of Kampo medicine. And in 1927, Kyushin Yumoto wrote his book *Nokan Igaku* (Superior Chinese Medicine) about the scientific research that had been done in the field of Kampo.

During the following year, 1928, many Kampo practitioners began to come out into the open and associations for Asian medicines were formed. Japan's Kampo Medicine Association was formally created in 1934 and began publishing a monthly newsletter called *Kampo To Kan'yaku* (Kampo and Kampo Medicine). The Association, a centralized organization for Kampo practitioners in Japan, was in existence until 1945.

The Japanese Medical Association was organized in 1936, and in 1938 the East Asian Medical Organization was created. The latter has been publishing the monthly *Kampo No Rinsho* (Clinical Kampo) since its founding.

The Japan Toyo Medical Association, created in 1950, is the largest medical organization in Japan today. Its main office is located at the Asian Medicine Research Center at Chiba University Medical Center.

Kampo Medicine in Present-Day Japan

Japanese Kampo medicine has undergone many changes. Despite its decline in the 19th century with the onset of orthodox medicine in Japan, there were still practitioners who continued their research in Kampo.

In 1955 their hard work was recognized and the practice of Kampo was revived in Japan. In the last ten years much knowledge of Kampo has been made public and many Kampo medicines and treatments are now accepted for insurance reimbursement by the government. This amounts to official acknowledgment that Kampo treatments are highly effective in curing many diseases.

"If you are weak, eat herbs,"—Romans 14: 2

CHAPTER 3

THE BASIC IDEA OF KAMPO

Kampo medicine is based on the theory that diseases arise due to a disharmony of bodily flow. By the same token, modern medicine frequently looks to the circulatory system.

Kampo medications are comprised of unrefined drugs which include not only herbs but also animal and mineral matter. Generally, each Kampo formula will contain several different drugs in specified amounts. These are mixed as directed by reference texts which were written and revised in accordance with previous usage. The unrefined drugs in Kampo work together through synergistic action to cure disease and restore the body's homeostasis. This is a unique characteristic of Kampo and is not found in orthodox medicine.

The first concern of the Kampo practitioner is the prevention of disease, thereby eliminating costly hospitalization. The aim of the treatment is not just to kill germs, but to correct conditions which permit disease to develop in the first place. Germs cannot attack strong, healthy organs successfully. This calls for a more sophisticated diagnosis and treatment than westerners are used to. As a rule, Kampo physicians spend much more time with each patient and make far more detailed examinations than western doctors.

Most westerners are surprised and delighted by this attention as evidenced in the case histories in Chapter 6. They are even more surprised at the final diagnosis which is couched in Asian terms, strange to American ears: yin and yang, ai, pure vital essences, the five elements and other cosmic forces, and meridians. What does it all mean?

What a westerner must understand is that these terms are in reality symbolic, even poetic, representations of fundamental natural forces. Oddly, this Asian frame of reference is amazingly precise in tracing the sources and course of disease even when measured by all the tools of modern science. In fact, Asian medicine is still well ahead of western medicine in treating the physical causes of mental disturbances.

New patients, under the care of a Kampo practitioner, are surprised when germs and viruses are not blamed for their ills. Instead, they are told that the problem lies deep in the organs that are weakened, and unable to resist attacks by toxins and bacteria. Killing the germs, therefore, only eliminates immediate symptoms and does not restore health. In fact, the powerful drugs usually administered only serve to weaken us further. The true cure is to correct the conditions which have left us vulnerable to illness. Germs cannot attack strong healthy organs.

Treating the Patient, Not the Symptoms

How do Kampo practitioners decide which organs are weakened? They rely on a host of basic indicators of health such as complexion, eye color, bodily odors, texture of the tongue, and pulse, plus painstaking interviewing, observing, listening, and feeling. The health history of the patient's family is also critical. The examiner even notes the patient's mood, and movements—the way he walks, talks, sits, and breathes.

Tactile examination includes traditional Asian pulse diagnosis, massage and palpation. The trained physician can detect six separate pulses on each wrist. Each of the twelve pulses indicates to him the condition of one of the vital organs. Past as well as current diseases sustained by the organ can be revealed by this method. This is a delicate art taking many years to master and requiring much practice.

Massaging the spinal column often indicates where a disease is located because the spinal nerves associated with the diseased organ are knotted and tight to the touch. Certain vital points along the meridians, called "alarm points," will be tender or even painful under acupressure when the related organ is diseased or weak.

Determining the nature and location of disease is only the beginning of Kampo diagnosis. To treat patients effectively with herbal mixtures, the physician must next make a "differential diagnosis" based on the symptoms. This is based on the direction in which the illness is moving. Symptoms sometimes seem to disappear during treatment. In actual fact, they have usually transformed and moved elsewhere. Halting treatment will only make it likely that the illness will return in the future. That is why the usual policy is to continue herbal treatment for some time after symptoms have disappeared. During treatment, herbal prescriptions are adjusted to conform to the everchanging symptomatic situation. Kampo physicians recognize that no two patients are alike in their reaction to disease or in their response to herbal medications. This is far cry from the habit of some doctors to prescribe a favorite wonder drug to every patient that comes their way!

What is Sho?

The concept of *Sho* is central to the study of Kampo. *Sho* is the basis for diagnosis and treatment in Kampo medicine. That is to say, the medical problem is identified, or named in terms of the treatment (Kampo prescription) prescribed. For example, when a patient is diagnosed as having *Kakkon-to-sho*, the doctor will prescribe *Kakkon-to*. Moreover, this is entirely different from the orthodox method of prescribing medication.

In this case, the In-yo (Yin-Yang) factors, *Kyo-sho* (weak resistance), *Jitsu-sho* (strong resistance), and *Chukan-sho* (middle resistance), are all taken into consideration.

A) Arriving at an *In-yo* diagnosis

1) When a patient comes in with symptoms such as acute fever, examination and categorization into one of the six stages of illness (*3 In-byo*, *3 Yo-byo*) follows.

3 In-byo In these 3 stages, the patient's resistant factors are weakened, as characterized by coldness in the hands and feet. However, chronic ailments, and non fever-producing illnesses, will be examined.

3 Yo-byo Patients categorized into any of these 3 stages still have resistant factors. Most have characteristics producing fever.

2) Symptoms of *Kan-sho* and *Netsu-sho*

Kan-sho. Bodily response to coldness. Since coldness is a characteristic of this *Sho*, the patient must warm himself by taking hot baths with raw drugs such as dried ginger administered to the water. There is no comparable treatment in orthodox medicine.

Netsu-sho Bodily response to fever. In cases of this sort, raw drugs must be administered to cool the body.

B) *Kyo-jitsu* Diagnosis

Jitsu-sho Robust constitution. The patient's physical nature, strength, body type, and muscle condition all must be taken into consideration.

Kyo-sho Deficient constitution. Lack of energy and vitality due to illness and physical characteristics such as small bones, weak muscles, and lack of strength all must be examined.

C) Special examination of Kampo medicine
(Illustrated Step-by-Step Explanation of Kampo Examinations)

D) Energy, Blood and Fluids diagnosed

Diseases are divided into three broad categories of energy, blood, and fluid condition. The examiner must distinguish the causative factors in the disease, such as the circulatory system, in which case the term Oketsu indicates blood-related problems.

CAVEAT: Before experimenting with herbs, readers are earnestly urged to give careful consideration to the nature of their particular health problem and to consult with a competent physician if in any doubt. This book should not be regarded as a substitute for professional medical treatment. While every care has been taken to ensure the accuracy of the contents, the author and the publisher cannot accept legal responsibility for any problem arising out of experimentation with the herbs described.

PART TWO

The Essential Life Force and the Art of Kampo

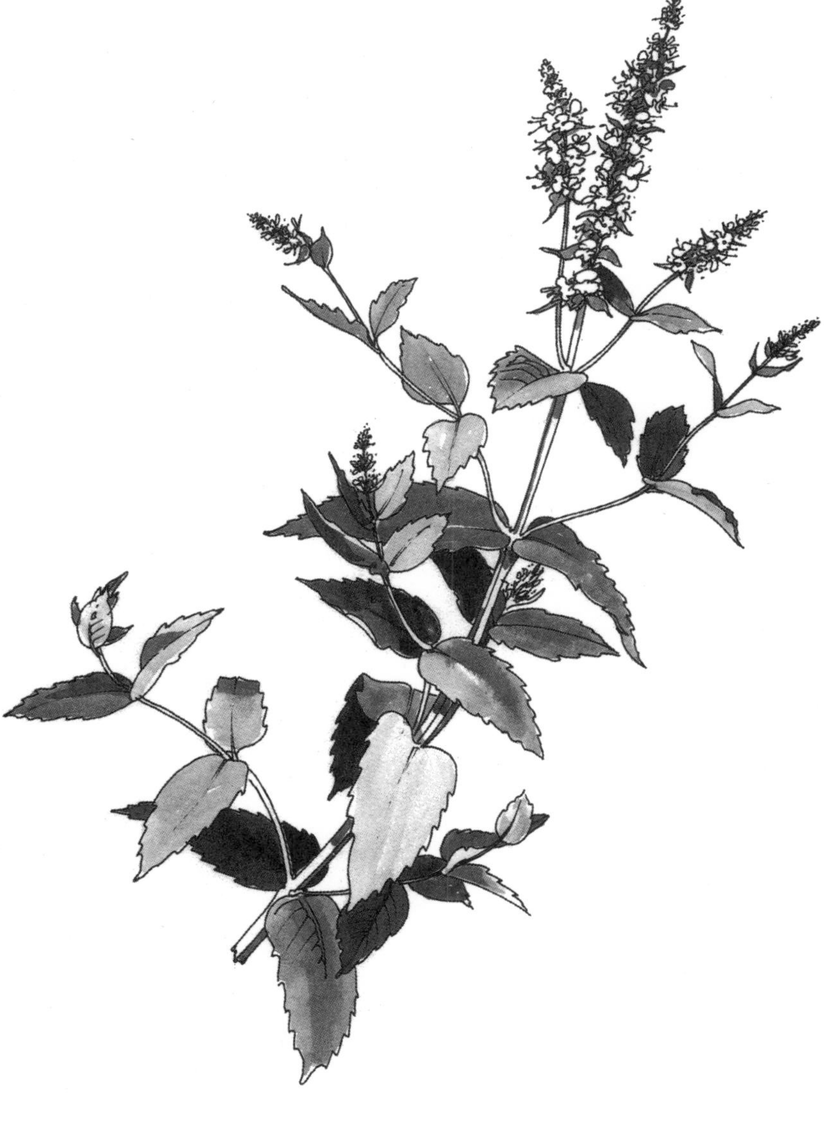

"There is a way of knowing, higher than human reason,"
—The Tao of Leadership

When Asia was opened to the West, a cultural revolution swept away many of our strongest traditions. Yet the art of herbal medicine was not swept away simply because its concept of preventive care was still valid even in the face of apparent western miracles. Now, finally, herbs are regaining recognition as a major medical resource. Perhaps it is also time we should re-examine the symbolism associated with them, to discover new truths in ancient folk wisdom.

The principles and premises of Asian herbalism are drawn directly from traditional Taoist philosophy and are, therefore, difficult for the average westerner to absorb easily. It would take much study for the uninitiated to absorb the remarkable insights which characterize the discipline.

What follows is only the first faltering step in understanding the basis of Kampo's medical concepts. However, folk wisdom reminds us that a long journey is only a succession of little steps.

QI

The major premise of Asian medical theory is that all forms of life in the universe are animated by an essential life force called *qi*. It is the quality, quantity and balance of your *qi* that determines your state of health and span of life. The key to maintaining optimal health is a natural and harmonious balance among the vital energies within the body. The most important factors affecting our quotient of *qi* are the food we consume and the air we breathe. That is why diet and breathing exercises are of such importance to the Asian practitioner.

Qi is also dependent on the ability of the stomach and lungs to absorb vital energy. If these are not functioning properly, the physician must correct this condition by prescribing a regimen of proper diet, exercise, breathing, and hygiene. Only when the physical problem has become so serious that it impairs the functioning of the vital organs and glands does the physician use herbal medications. The *qi* in the plant, nature's remedy, goes directly to the organ and gland in need of revival.

Qi is but one of four bodily humors, but is by far the most important one. The others are blood, fluid, and vital essence. Vital essence is stored in the glands straddling the kidneys, and released into the bloodstream as needed. It is also found in the spermatazoa of the male, and the ova in the female.

YIN and YANG

Yin and *yang* are already familiar to Western ears. They are central to Taoist philosophy as well as to herbal medicine. The balance between these two primordial cosmic forces is the key factor in all natural phenonema and life processes.

Yin represents the negative, passive force. It is female in nature and is symbolized by water. *Yang* symbolizes the positive, active force. It is male in nature and is represented by fire.

Yin and *yang* are mutually dependent. Therefore, the ideal state of all nature, including a person's health, is a harmonious balance between the two.

The perfect *yin yang* balance is often disturbed in life. For example, during the winter when cold *yin* forces dominate, the body requires extra warming *yang* energy. When the body fills with excess *yang* energy driving out *yin* to the point of deficiency, then cooling *yin* medicine is prescribed. Usually, the body itself adjusts this balance. When it does not, a special diet or medicine is prescribed. To be successful, Kampo practitioners must master a delicate balancing act.

THE FIVE ELEMENTS

How do Asian herbalists explain the interdependence of the various organs? By using symbols: Wood, Fire, Earth, Metal, and Water. (Wood represents the liver; Fire, the heart; Earth, the spleen; Metal, the lungs; and Water, the kidneys.) Wood burns to generate Fire; Fire produces ashes, which generate Earth; Earth generates Metal which, when molten, becomes like water; and Water promotes growth of plants, thereby generating Wood. Since each vital organ belongs to one of the Five Elements they can be used as code words to bodily functions. Amazingly, to western minds, this exotic system actually duplicates the findings of modern medical research to perfection, although there is not enough space in this book to demonstrate this fully. However, it must be pointed out that in one field at least, mental illness, this symbolic method actually gives superior results in diagnosis and treatment!

THE MERIDIANS

Western medical science itself has nothing matching the meridians spoken of by herbal practitioners. The most common western view is that these are fibers of the autonomous nervous system. But Asian practitioners deny this, pointing out that *qi* travels about the body where there are no nerve fibers and that meridians, the great connecting system of the body, only manifest themselves functionally, not physically. Hard to dispute when this is part of the basis for acupuncture, now accepted in the West.

Apparently, there are a total of fifty-nine meridians in the body, of which twelve dominate the others. Each of the main meridians represents a biological energy system centered around one of the twelve vital organs. Acupuncturists know these meridians well, and so do adepts of Taoist breathing techniques. Kampo doctors also know how to use herbs to stimulate the main meridians as well as the bloodstream. Amazingly, this enables the herbs to promote general vitality at the same time they are improving the health of an individual organ. This long-term benefit is one western doctors now appreciate, but still cannot understand.

"The Lord hath created medicine out of the earth, and he that is wise will not abhor them,"—Apocrypha, Ecclesiasticus 34.4

CHAPTER 1

THE POPULARITY AND VALIDITY OF KAMPO

Why is Kampo medicine receiving so much attention at the present time? There are many reasons for the rise in interest surrounding Kampo.

Side Effects in Orthodox Medicine

In recent years, the incidence of certain diseases such as tuberculosis and pneumonia has decreased due to the discovery by orthodox medicine of drugs which cure the infections that cause these diseases. However, it has been found that these same drugs tend to cause abnormalities in elderly patients and those with circulatory ailments. Tragically, orthodox medicine does nothing about this.

Many success stories in orthodox medicine fail to report the side effects that often occur, particularly if long term use of a given drug is involved. The mere mention of penicillin deaths or thalidomide deformities can send a shock wave through the medical community, which is now painfully aware of the Jekyll-Hyde character of many of today's wonder drugs.

Recently there were reports of cases such as that involving the Ciba-Geigy corporation in Japan. Not long after Ciba-Geigy began to distribute a new sedative for the treatment of arthritis and rheumatism, it was found that the drug could cause stomach ulcers, blood diseases, and even death.

The dangers of this drug were reported worldwide, sparking an instant reaction. Many countries began an immediate investigation of this and other drugs. In Japan, the furor resulted in stricter drug regulations and in the revision of all instructions for medicinal use to insure safer dosages.

The greater result of this tragedy, however, was that many people lost confidence in doctors and prescriptions. In fact, there was a marked increase in people who, despite having gone to orthodox physicians, still have not been able to learn what ails them, or who are unable to use orthodox medicine due to the severity of side-effects.

Some orthodox medical researchers are still skeptical about the efficacy of Kampo medicine. They request scientific proof of actual improvement without harmful side-effects in patients treated with Kampo.

Many Advantages

Treatment by a Kampo physician does have many advantages. By stressing prevention, it helps eliminate last-minute, costly trips to the hospital. It helps the patient discover the true sources of illness, allowing the patient to vary diet and lifestyle to build good health. Best of all, it relies on safe herbs instead of dangerous, synthetic drugs and painful surgery. That is why there is a movement around the world to blend this ancient art with the best of modern science to offer a "New Medicine" for the sick.

Kampo's Effect on Cancer

Kampo has received the attention of researchers world-wide, especially in herbal cures for cancer, since a 1984 meeting. Since herbs seem to be of universal value in treating all diseases, it is reasonable to assume that somewhere there is an herb that will cure cancer. (Herbalists predict that soon 1,400 or more rare plants containing effective new remedies will be found in tropical rain forests.)

Many people know the Rosy Periwinkle, *Catharanthus roseus*, as a small pot plant with showy pink or white flowers. It was used for hundreds of years in the tropics as an anti-diabetic. In the 1950's a medical research laboratory in Canada discovered that it also could halt leukemia. After many more years of testing, it was found that one of its alkaloids, vincristine, was the key. Another alkaloid, vinblastine, now produces a remission rate of 80% in Hodgkin's disease. Other types of cancer are now being halted or cured by these drugs.

Spurred by the World Health Organization (WHO), scientists in countries around the world are feverishly testing thousands of plants for new cures. Many plants already show promise: The American Mandrake, *Podophyllum peltatum*, used by Penobscot Indians to treat malignant tumors. In India, the Himalayan *Podophyllum hexandrum*. The East African shrub *Maytenus gratius*. The American Meadow Rue, *Thalictrum dasycarpum*. The Chinese Plum-yew, *Cephalotaxus fortuni*. The bark of the *Croton lechleri*, found deep in the South American rain forest. And the bark of the *Jacaranda caucana*, used to treat leukemia. Every day there are new discoveries. The dainty little Bloodroot, *Sanguinaria canadensis*, has now been confirmed as having value in treating malignant tumors.

Seventeenth International Medical Association (1984)

The participants at the meeting of the Seventeenth International Internal Medicine

Association in Kyoto, Japan, included representatives from 56 countries, who spoke on the theme of "Internal Medicine of the East and West—A View of Tomorrow." Reports on 41 cases of clinical use of Kampo throughout the world were presented in two symposia on traditional and Asian medicine.

"Symposium 9: Traditional Asian Medicine" included presentations by Dr. Katsuyoshi Terasawa of Japan on the "Secession of Steroids Produced by Kampo Medicine," and by Hiromichi Yasui on "The Effects of Asian and Modern Western Medicine."

Dr. Yasui, also of Japan, is a Kampo researcher at the Kitasato Research Center. He is noted for his *Facts about Kampo*, which is based on case studies using Kampo therapy alone rather than cases in which both Kampo and orthodox medicine were used.

At "Satellite Symposium 8: Traditional Medicine," 34 cases of actual clinical use of traditional Asian medicine were reported. The highlight of this gathering was the introduction of research equipment used to check the validity of Kampo.

The amount of time currently devoted to such research demonstrates that there are still large numbers of physicians around the world who are puzzled by the inability of allopathic medicine to find the causes of many chronic diseases as well as to discover appropriate treatments for them. It also demonstrates that there is growing world recognition and interest in Kampo.

The New Medicine in Developing Countries

Interest in herbal medicine is increasing world wide at a rapid rate out of simple necessity. For years, the World Health Organization has been working tirelessly to incorporate a knowledge of healing plants into the health systems of developing countries. For the great majority of the world's poor, a local healer represents the only medical care available. The hospital or the clinic is often far away, understaffed, and a frightening place.

However, a new era started when the 30th World Health Assembly adopted a resolution (WHA30.49) calling for a rebirth of the medicine of the past. It urged interested governments to give "adequate importance to the utilization of their traditional systems of medicine with appropriate regulations as suited to their national health systems." The result? Almost unanimous acceptance world wide. In many instances, appropriate legislation was passed immediately. Alternative health systems, once scorned, are now backed by official government agencies in hundreds of countries.

In China, where herbal medicine is so much a part of its history, its practitioners are now accepted as equals by western-trained doctors. Acupuncture, massage, and herbal medicine are being used in every province, combined with the best western techniques. Over a million "barefoot" doctors now bear witness to the value of the "New Medicine" using the best of both worlds, East and West.

There is also an historic new scientific journal in China—the Chinese Journal of Integrated Traditional and Western Medicine—published every two months since

1980 that is promoting cooperation among all those with a stake in improving the quality of health care.

Japan, I am proud to say, is using sophisticated research to help scientists understand how certain ancient practices do succeed where modern medicine may not. Exciting breakthroughs have also been made in analyzing the active ingredients of decoctions and ointments made from plants which have been proven to possess curative properties. The Russians, too, are far ahead of the rest of the modern world in such studies because they never developed a contempt for folk medicine.

Similar research is being carried on in the poorer nations as well. One example among many is the Biochemical Research Unit on Traditional and Herbal Medicine in Mexico City. This unit is engaged in intensive pharmacological, chemical and botanical research into plants which were known to the Aztecs, the Mayans, and other earlier civilizations. Scientists here make use of liquid and gas chromatography, magnetic resonance, and even radio isotopes to separate and identify the active ingredients of healing herbs. The findings are stored in a computerized data bank which can be referred to under many headings: botanical names, popular names, the methods of use, the part of the plant used, and the diseases treated. A rich treasure house of folk wisdom!

The Vietnamese are also making remarkable progress despite a slow start. They have not only had to face endemic tropical diseases but also extreme medical and surgical demands resulting from decades of war. As a result, families there are being encouraged to grow at least a dozen of the 58 common "family medicine" herbs of the countryside. The government now buys most of its medicinal raw materials from these gardens so that the villagers now have both improved health care and a source of badly needed extra income. In recent years, a massive effort in Vietnam's network of new research institutes, studying local plant remedies, has discovered more than forty new drugs for disorders as varied as high blood pressure, rheumatism, hepatitis, goiter, allergy and shock. Other countries encouraging the production of medical herbs in a similar manner are Bangladesh, Rwanda, and Thailand.

In Africa, where expenditure on health care is the lowest in the world, farmers and nomads are forced to depend on the medicinal plants that they know about and can find. However, their native healers do serve a long apprenticeship and manage to arrive at a remarkable botanical knowledge of local plants, their uses and properties. All this knowledge, unfortunately, is in grave danger of being lost as increasing human and livestock populations put more pressure on natural vegetation.

One man who understands this is Dr. Herbert Ushewokuaze, Zimbabwe's Minister of Health. In 1980, soon after independence, he formed a National Traditional Healer's Association and put its members to work as part of the Zimbabwe's National Health Service.

Six of the healers told him they could reduce surgical operations by 80%, using herbal medicine!

His proud answer: "*African medicine is part and parcel of our culture. Previous white governments tended to discredit and scorn our traditional healers, portraying them as evil by calling them witch doctors. Now we are calling them back to their rightful place.*"

In Pakistan, traditional medicine, known as Unani Tibb, is also accepted as a state system alongside modern medicine. It has 36,000 practitioners, or *hakims*, who are graduates of the nine Tibbi medical schools. They reach all of the rural areas in Pakistan as well as the cities. A National Council regulates and maintains standards.

India, too, has a very elaborate system of traditional medicine with 900 hospitals and 14,000 dispensaries. However, the traditional healers are still subordinated to doctors educated in western-style practice and who discourage the older Ayurvedic theories. The good news is that research into traditional herbal healing is increasing in India today. This depth of research into the healing power of plants is expected to be a strong influence in western medicine in the future. In India alone, many helpful drugs are being discovered daily, offering hope for sufferers from leprosy, dysentery, hepatitis, and soon we hope, from cancer and AIDS.

Of course, all new discoveries must be carefully evaluated in modern laboratories. People must be taught how to use them properly. Synthesis of the basic compounds is urgent also if we are to protect ourselves from the over-collection of the world's precious healing plants. Many are already endangered. And, tragically, controls are slow to be enacted by government bodies.

Another difficulty is that some local practitioners are wary of western ways and do not wish to share their knowledge with us. An even greater problem we must face soon is that the wholesale destruction of habitats is seriously endangering not only those plants we know and use, but also those which could be useful in the future. Experts are so concerned that one spokesman, Chiang Mai of Thailand, called for an international program for the conservation of medicinal plants.

Where are large supplies of medicinal herbs to be found today? One of the last remaining sources, not yet overworked, is in Malaysia.

In the three decades or more since Malaysia's independence, Kuala Lumpur has become a major source of herbal medicines. Herbs are obtainable in large quantities from more than a hundred major distributors, and from the city's crowded spice shops and street markets. Popular choices are drugs to increase one's vitality and sex drive, regulate blood sugar levels for diabetics, reduce high blood pressure, and cure the flu. The University of Malaysia has established a *Rimbu Iimu* (Knowledge Forest) to grow and display valuable herbs, and has also established a research laboratory to study their action in the human body. Western scholars are now investigating this treasure trove of medicinal herbs with enthusiasm.

What About America?

The picture is changing rapidly in the U.S., even in this drug-oriented culture. New ideas are winning acceptance as this is written.

One dramatic example is the bestselling, true story by Norman Cousins, "The Anatomy of An Illness." It is one of the most widely reprinted and discussed medical accounts in recent years. Briefly, it is the story of the author's resolve to beat his own "terminal illness" and how he succeeded. The concept of patient responsibility for his own well-being is presented in winning terms and struck a responsive chord in readers around the world. People once dependent on a large medical establishment now realize that their state of health rests on their own shoulders. (A decision hastened by the rapidly escalating cost of professional medical care.)

Americans in particular have become aerobic-exercise addicts and are slimming down, giving up tobacco, eating more healthy foods, and discovering herbs. They now appreciate the Chinese maxim, "Good food is the best medicine." After all, aren't such common garden substances as almonds, garlic, cucumbers, ginger, mint, pepper, walnuts, and sunflower seeds the basis of Chinese herbal medicine?

Another reason for this common-sense trend to healthy living is that, tragically, the medical establishment itself has oftentimes become a threat to our health. The side effects of powerful, synthesized drugs have become so devastating that a new word has been coined for the epidemic—*latrogenesis.* It is now a major topic of discussion at medical conferences as doctors search for a way to deal with the alarming side-effects of drugs. No greater popular fallacy exists about medicine than that a drug is like an arrow that can be shot at a particularized target. Its actual effect is more like a shower of porcupine quills. Even a steady diet of aspirin can cause internal bleeding, intensify arthritis, and in extreme cases, can be lethal! (Particularly notorious side-effects are congenital defects caused by thalidomide cancers of the vagina and uterine cervix in daughters of women who took DES, or diethylstilbestrol, during their pregnancy many years earlier.)

In Sweden, in August 1979, the government had to acknowledge its medical mistakes by putting into force an insurance plan to compensate patients harmed by prescription drugs!

In the U.S. today, there is even a high-volume debate over the value of synthesized vitamins and mineral supplements. The National Academy of Sciences (NAS) recently issued a report rejecting the idea of using such supplements to make up for deficiencies in the diet or to prevent disease. It pointed out, in addition, that megadoses of vitamins A, D, and B_6 could cause serious side effects.

No wonder that there has been a sudden interest in ancient cultures and renewed respect for them and for their folk remedies. People are having their eyes opened to the important social function fulfilled in other cultures by herbalists and other practitioners of traditional medicine who value human dignity as opposed to modern doctors who treat the disease but seem to have lost sight of the patient.

Indeed, plant compounds have won a far greater acceptance than most of us realize. Medicinal plants are not a thing of the past. Far from it! In recent years, natural products accounted for almost half of all the prescriptions dispensed in community pharmacies in the U.S.

The winds of change are sweeping through the West as the oldest, safest medicine in the world stages a comeback.

"Green Medicine is being born again,"—Anthony Huxley

CHAPTER 2

THE FASCINATION OF KAMPO

Many western medical students who originally went to Japan to study such methods as acupuncture and moxibustion, both of which seem to be gaining popularity outside Asia, are now becoming interested in Kampo.

One of the reasons for this fascination with Japanese medicine is the nation's intriguing longevity statistic. Why do the people of Japan have a longer average lifespan than those of other countries? One theory is that it might have something to do with the Japanese diet which is centered around rice, vegetables and fish. Along with that, we must consider Japanese health care in general.

With the latter in mind, I took the opportunity of interviewing three western exchange students at the Kitasato University Affiliated Asian Medicine Research Center in Tokyo. All three are studying under the direction of Dr. Yasuo Otsuka, the leading authority on Kampo medicine in Japan. By talking with the students rather than the teacher, I was able to get more of an "outsider's" viewpoint, for until recently, these people had been completely unfamiliar with the methods and effects of Kampo.

◇ ◇ ◇

Peter Townsend, age 29
Mr. Townsend was born in New Zealand and has lived in Japan for the past five years.

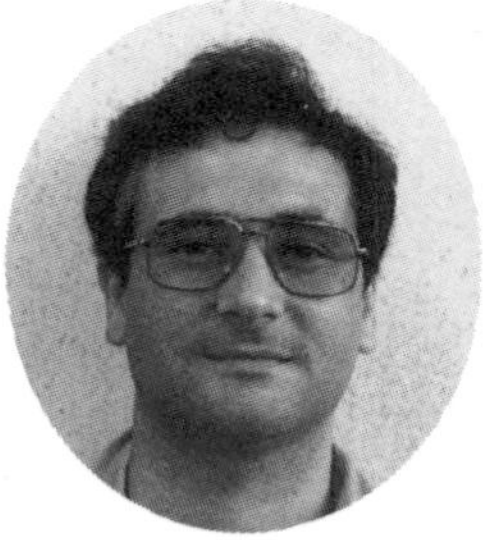

Q. How did you become interested in the field of Kampo?

A. I used to work for a pharmaceutical import-export company. I had to know which medication was appropriate for what symptom. There were no texts for looking up the products so I was on my own but I gained a pretty full knowledge of which medicines were good for building stamina, which were good for the digestive system, and so on. This is the sort of information that is needed in the field of Kampo.

Q. In your handling of pharmaceuticals, were you able to gain some knowledge of Kampo?
A. Yes. We used to import from countries such as Korea, and I often heard mention of Kampo. All I knew then was that the medicines were a mixture of various herbs. I was used to orthodox medicine and had never heard of Kampo before. But it seemed to me that it made sense to mix herbs that were good for the body and use them for medicinal purposes.

Q. Isn't the mixing of herbs in Kampo quite different from the way orthodox medicines are produced?
A. Yes, it is, and I think the idea of mixing various natural herbs is a good one. Orthodox medical theory focuses on finding medicine to bring down a fever, and on developing antibiotics to fight against infection. Kampo has a different approach. If a person gets a fever, Kampo practitioners try to predict whether the fever will continue to rise or go down, and whether it needs to be brought down immediately or gradually. Furthermore, the human organism is very complex, and one person's body may react differently from another's. For that reason, each Kampo medication is individually prescribed.

Q. When did you begin studying Kampo?
A. I began in December 1980, almost as soon as I came to Japan. Because I didn't speak Japanese, my first step was to attend a language school for nine months.

Q. Did you have much difficulty studying Japanese?
A. I thought studying kanji, the Chinese writing, was the hardest part. All Kampo terms are written in kanji, and most of those characters are old forms that are no longer used. I think it was only because of my interest in Kampo that I was able to learn all that difficult kanji.

Q. Since Kampo is different from the kind of medicine you are used to, did you have any trouble understanding it?
A. I was able to absorb the concept of Kampo quite easily, but the next stage was very difficult. That is the method used to prescribe Kampo. There's a special way in which to examine each condition and prescribe the appropriate Kampo mixture.

In Kampo medicine, you see, one must be able to use many different kinds of examinations in order to grasp the total picture of a patient's health. The secret of Kampo is to master Sho, to be able to find the strong and weak points of the patient's body. That type of analysis is unique to Kampo.

Q. What do you find most unusual about the theory of Sho?

A. Until I learned about Sho, I couldn't understand why the prescriptions for Mr. A and Mr. B had to be different. In orthodox medicine, you would give the same prescription for the same symptom, even if the patients are two different people. Not so with Kampo.

Q. Then it's through the use of Sho that the prescriptions are individualized?
A. Yes, but even a prescription for the same person can change. For example, when the patient is very weak, one medication will be given, but as he gains a little more strength, the medication may be changed. In addition to prescribing medication to fit the disease, Kampo also fits the medication to the physical condition of a patient's body.

Q. It is often said that modern medical treatments are carried out without concern for the patient. How do you feel about this statement? Is Kampo any different?
A. Of course it's very important to examine the patient's symptoms even when using modern medical treatments. In Kampo, however, the patient's complaints are the main factors in determining treatment. Kampo works best when the practitioner really listens to a patient's complaints. All this close attention helps put the patient at ease psychologically, so there's rarely that feeling of neglect or rejection that many patients in the west have mentioned. Maybe that's why western medicine is now making an effort to re-emphasize the psychological role of the doctor in healing.

Q. Are you saying that orthodox medicine is systemized? Impersonal?
A. Unfortunately, yes. For instance, if a patient went to a western-trained doctor for treatment of hysteria with accompanying stomach pains, because of the patient's mental state, the stomach pains would probably be ignored. In Kampo, every complaint the patient has will be thoroughly examined. Orthodox medicine is divided into distinct areas such as psychology, or internal and external medicine, and you have to go to a doctor who specializes in your type of symptom. This is nonsense. The body and mind are all part of the same person, and I think basically all disorders should be treated together.

Q. Listening to you speak, I can tell you know the exact difference between orthodox and Kampo medicine.
A. Yes, I think so. One time I developed tympanitis, an ear infection, which produced a slight fever. I took a Kampo formula called *Kakkon-to* for a week and was cured.

Q. Did you prepare your own prescription?
A. Yes. *Kakkon-to* is one of the first Kampo medicines I learned to prepare.

Q. Prescribing Kampo is very complex. Did you have trouble learning it?
A. Remembering which herbs are mixed together is difficult. But once I learn

why a mixture is effective or why certain Kampos are mixed, I find it easier to remember and very interesting. Ginseng, you know, is widely used in Kampo. However, western doctors fail to recognize that ginseng is effective for both hypo- and hypertension.

Q. Do you mean that in Kampo ginseng is used to treat completely opposite conditions? That ought to be of interest to people studying orthodox medicine.
A. I agree. A Russian named Breckman explains this theory by saying "adapt to the generic." This means that the medicine itself should lower hypertension and also increase the flow of blood in hypotension. I don't think any orthodox medical treatment has this type of effectiveness.
Q. Isn't this a difficult theory to explain?
A. That's where the idea of Sho comes in. No matter how effective a Kampo medicine may be, if it is not appropriate for that particular individual's Sho, it is of no use. That's why Kampo practitioners take plenty of time to examine the entire Sho.

Q. Do you feel that there's a great difference between Kampo and modern medicine?
A. Besides the question of effectiveness, the market-life of Kampo medicine differs greatly from that of orthodox medicine. Western drugs appear on the market and often disappear within five years. Many Kampo remedies, however, have been in existence for thousands of years.

Q. Can you give an example of such Kampo?
A. DAIO (*rheum officinale*) is one. It is used during blood transfusions.

Q. Kampo is beginning to get some recognition from the European medical establishment. When you go back to New Zealand, do you have any plans for informing people there about Kampo?
A. Yes, I have. I am thinking of translating the Shang Han Lun medical text into English. Then, when I return to New Zealand, I can use it to help people learn about Kampo.

◇

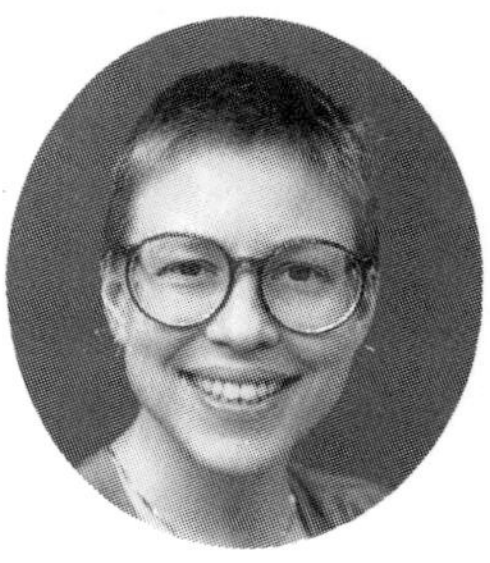

Gleson Soriano, age 36
Ms. Soriano was born in Virginia, U.S.A., and has been living in Japan for six years.

Q. What are you studying here in Japan?
A. I am studying acupuncture and moxibustion at a school in Yotsuya. I never knew about acupuncture or moxa treatments before coming to Japan and have found Japanese medicine to be fascinating.

Q. Why did you decide to study Japanese medicine?
A. My mother died from liver problems. I remember her saying that she had spent her entire savings in the course of a year because she had to undergo one examination after another while she was in the hospital. It was expensive, but they needed to do those diagnostic tests.

Q. Your mother must have suffered much pain.
A. She did, but there seemed no alternative. At that time I accepted orthodox medicine as the most scientific and efficient treatment. As the only treatment, in fact. But I also felt something was missing, and that suspicion stuck in my mind.

Q. What do you think was missing?
A. Let me explain it this way. When I began studying Japanese medicine, I noticed a great difference. I think what the orthodox medical field lacks is kindness and individual concern. Modern medicine seems to regard people as machines, or mere organisms. A prescription "menu" has been created and established for each disorder, and the doctor merely says, "For this case, let's prescribe this medicine."
In traditional Japanese medicine, however, it's believed that although the symptoms may appear in one place in the body, the cause might be located somewhere else. Therefore, the entire body is examined. On top of that, it is recognized that each person is different, with his own individual variations. Consequently, each person is treated individually.

Q. Can you explain one of these procedures in detail?
A. When someone comes in complaining of stomach trouble, it is treated by pressure points in the hands and feet. I was surprised to learn this myself when I started studying acupuncture and moxibustion. This is understandable if you know that Japanese medicine aims to harmonize the flow of the entire body. But I was not aware of such a theory and so it was a totally new concept to me.

Q. So your studies of acupuncture and moxibustion turned you toward the study of Kampo?
A. Yes. I began learning Kampo after a year's study of acupuncture and moxibustion. I've always been aware of folk herbal remedies, such as drinking mint tea for sinus conditions, but Kampo is different from that. Kampo is a mixture of raw medicines that work naturally, from within.

And there are so many variations of Kampo. Even if several patients all have similar conditions, the prescription for each may be different. On top of that, the same person's prescription will be altered with every change in his condition. Kampo medicines are custom tailored and designed to work for the individual.

Q. Have you ever tried Kampo yourself?

A. Yes, I've taken *Kami-shoyo-san* when I was feeling irritable and unwell. A researcher at the university recommended it.

Q. *Kami-shoyo-san* is often used in the special Kampo examination called *Oketsu*, isn't it?
A. Yes. I was told that my irritability came from *Oketsu*, but at the time, I couldn't understand that. When I first saw the label on the *Kami-shoyo-san* bottle telling what it was most effective for, I didn't think it applied to me. Surprisingly, however, it did. It worked so well that I immediately became interested in Kampo. It fascinated me to picture all the many, varied ingredients in *Kami-shoyo-san* working inside my body. I found this first experience with Kampo quite overwhelming.

Q. Did you brew your own medication?
A. Happily I didn't have to. It came in handy capsule form. I found out later that this Kampo used to be brewed in water and then drunk. But because of the long time it takes to brew *Kami-shoyo-san*, and the strong odor it produces, there aren't many people who make it themselves nowadays.

Kami-shoyo-san includes such herbs as Chinese thoroughwax, poria cocos, Chinese licorice, skin of the peony, jasmine, ginger, and peppermint. At one time, all those herbs had to be brewed daily. It must have been quite a job.

Q. How did *Kami-shoyo-san* taste?
A. It had an interesting flavor. It gave me a feeling of being at one with nature. I feel that my studies in Kampo have become second nature since I tried Kampo myself. There are texts that explain exactly what will result from taking which Kampo. It's all true actually. The doctors have treated so many people for such a long time and carefully recorded all the data, that they can now predict the results quite accurately. Kampo practitioners don't treat diseases, they treat the patient.

Q. Is it true, then, that Kampo is quite different from orthodox medicine which puts the emphasis on finding the cause of a disease and ridding the body of it?
A. I think it's like climbing a mountain. Someone who has weak legs will take an easier path. But someone who has confidence in climbing will attempt a steep path. Kampo sets up a program according to each person's physical condition. In that sense, Kampo considers people first.

Q. Are you planning to use Kampo in your work?
A. I'd like to further my studies of Kampo, then go back to the United States and try to help people who are suffering from illnesses that orthodox medicine can't seem to cure.

Pamela E. Langley, age 30
Ms. Langley was born in Australia

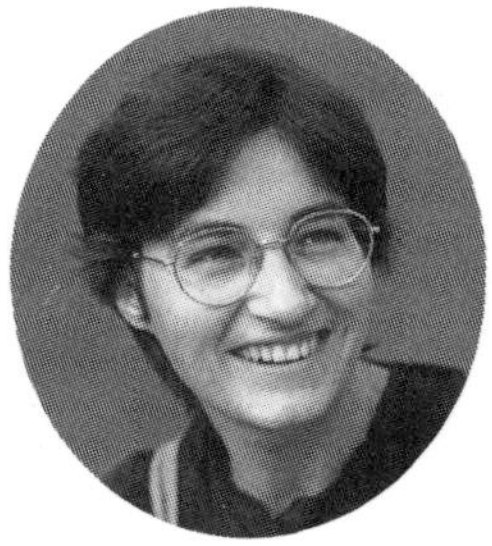

Q. Your Japanese is very good. How long have you been here in Japan?
A. Seven years. Before coming here 1 studied Japanese and Asian culture at a university in Australia. It made me decide I wanted to see present-day Japan, and so I came.

Q. What kind of work do you do?
A. I'm a translator. Japanese to English and English to Japanese. I am also studying Kampo, and I enjoy that more than anything.

Q. Do you mean you're enjoying Kampo more than your college specialty?
A. At first I was studying acupuncture. Gradually I began putting more emphasis on Kampo, and how I'm studying it exclusively.

Q. How did you become interested in acupuncture and Kampo?
A. I hurt my back after coming to Japan. I went to a university hospital, but I didn't get well. Then a friend told me about acupuncture. After two or three treatments, my back problems were cured. That's how I became interested in acupuncture and began my studies.

Q. How does acupuncture work?
A. When a needle is inserted in the appropriate acupoint (pressure point), the patient's pain can be stopped. Don't you think that's fascinating?

Q. So your own experience with acupuncture made you want to learn it. Did you study it long?
A. Two or three years. I studied at a clinic in Yoyogi, Tokyo. I found the examination method used in acupuncture and Japanese medicine to be very interesting. It's a special kind of theory.

Q. Would you explain that?
A. Orthodox medicine performs examinations with a straightforward approach, but it has its blind side. In Japanese medicine, you examine the entire body. I wanted to look into the differences between these two concepts. When I watched a Kampo practitioner performing an examination, I noticed him listening attentively to the patient's explanation of her symptoms. The practitioner did not act annoyed or impatient. This may sound easy, but actually it isn't.

Q. Good communication between the doctor and patient can make a big difference. Do you know how this detailed form of communication originated? Do students of Kampo question this system?

A. This is a concept found only in Kampo, and I don't totally understand it yet. Just as I still haven't mastered the concept of "energy, blood, and fluids."

Q. It's an ancient Chinese way of thinking. Can you compare it with the philosophy of the West?
A. When I was attending Champbella University, a professor told us, "In medicine, you have to go back to nature." These words have great significance for me now that I'm studying Kampo. Instead of prescribing scientifically calculated medications as in orthodox medicine, Kampo prescribes natural things such as grasses and bark. Some of these remedies are food we are accustomed to eating, so you can see that Kampo medicine is a natural medicine.

Q. Have you ever taken a Kampo treatment?
A. Yes, I have. I enjoy bike riding and ride my bicycle everywhere I go, usually about 14 km (8.75 miles) per day. Recently my knees began to hurt, probably from riding too much. I not only couldn't ride my bike, but I wasn't even able to walk very well. I began searching for a Kampo that would help me. I found *Boi-ogi-to* and tried it. After I had taken it for three or four days, the severe pain in my knees disappeared completely. I had truly experienced the effectiveness of natural grasses and bark.

Boi-ogi-to is a mixture of sinomenium acutum, ginger, giant jujube tree, and Chinese licorice. It's effective for rheumatism, arthritis, nephritis, and conditions of the knee joints.

I had another experience with Kampo, too. When I was breast-feeding my baby, I began to develop symptoms like those of menopause—dizziness and irritability—and my body stopped making milk. This time I took *Hochu-ekki-to*. This Kampo is effective for symptoms such as loss of energy after an illness, heaviness in the arms and legs, and unpleasant aftertaste. That was exactly the way I was feeling, and again the Kampo brought relief.

Q. I've often heard that when you see an orthodox doctor for menopause symptoms (heaviness in the head and poor health), you'll often be told that there is nothing wrong with you physically, that it's a psychological problem. Has that been your experience?
A. Yes. But I believe that in Kampo medicine the doctor and the patient work together to cure the body of its disorder. This is why I'd like to further my studies of Kampo, with an emphasis on Kampo for women.

Unlike men, women have monthly cycles that affect bodily conditions, work, and even human relations. In orthodox medicine, menstrual irregularities or cramps are often considered a sign of weakness. On that point alone, we can see how Kampo medicine is working for humankind. I would like to let more people know about the effectiveness of Kampo. That is my greatest wish.

". . . Kampo now meets every test of modern medicine . . ."

—Akira Tsumura

CHAPTER 3

HERBAL MEDICINE GOES HI-TECH

The capsules referred to by Gleson Soriano in previous pages are just one key to the rapid growth of Kampo in Japan.

In any traditional Chinese herbal shop throughout the world today you get a feeling that little has changed in the course of thousands of years. You are greeted by rows of worn wooden drawers, a heavy teak counter, crude balance scales and an abacus, choppers and grinders identical with those in the ancient scrolls, and the age-old varieties of crude herbs themselves.

Why hasn't someone modernized the ancient art of herbal healing? Why hasn't someone refined and purified the healing ingredients and concentrated them to produce modern medications in capsules and ampules? Why is it still up to the patient to mix the ingredients, prepare tea or broth as carefully as he can to the proper strength, and then down it manfully despite what is often a bitter taste?

In Japan, we asked ourselves those questions a long time ago and began a painstaking scientific examination of all the traditional herbal remedies. Today, we can truly state that herbal medicine has come of age. Kampo prescriptions are now virtually indistinguishable from any other modern drug. At Ibaragi, Japan, Tsumura & Co. has developed and consolidated the most modern research and development center in the field. The five institutes based there are leaders in the "New Medicine" being actively promoted worldwide by the World Health Organization. (Perhaps because the head of the WHO is a Japanese, Director General Dr. Hiroshi Nakajima.)

In Ibaragi, every aspect of pharmaceutical science is being explored in the five Tsumura divisions: The Research Institute for Pharmacology, the Institute for Molecular Genetics, the Research Department of Quality Control and Evaluation, and the Department of Technology.

The result? For the last several decades Kampo medications have been accepted by doctors and hospitals throughout Japan, fully accredited by the government health authorities. Hundreds of thousands of patients have taken Kampo remedies without realizing it, as they now meet every test of modern medicine and are refined to look much like any other medication.

Kampo capsules are so much easier to take than the original village herbal concoctions. And they are carefully measured to the exact dosage needed.

One by one, we are discovering the active ingredients in ancient remedies and synthesizing them in the laboratory. We have documented the effectiveness of Kampo medicinals in fields where western drugs have been almost useless: viral infections and allergies, asthma, chronic hepatitis, ulcers, and cirrhosis of the liver. Kampo medicines are also now highly recommended for diseases of the elderly where more gentle prescriptions are called for. Vitamins, too, we find are most easily and naturally metabolized when administered through herbal sources.

Another finding is that Kampo components react synergistically in the human body. Most contain between four and eighteen different crude drug extracts. We've found and reported in medical literature that the interaction of ingredients in Kampo prescriptions gives far better results than you would expect by simply adding up the benefits of each individual ingredient.

Each one has a synergistic, or catalytic, effect on all the others, increasing their effectiveness, working together to restore the patient's entire physical well being slowly, naturally—miraculously!

No wonder we find our work so exciting. Our research divisions right now are working full time, using the latest techniques of molecular biology, and chemical compound synthesis, to discover new chemical compounds that may soon heal all cancers, AIDS, and other diseases of the modern age.

CHAPTER 4

CURED BY KAMPO

Many Westerners living in Japan have tried Kampo as a treatment for numerous illnesses, and have found it to be highly effective. Here are some of their experiences, told exactly as reported. For those readers who want more than just a case history, we have provided scientific definitions and explanations of the various concepts used in the field.

◇ ◇ ◇

Case Study #1: John Branun, Age 30

- **Born in Manchester, England**
- **Has lived in Japan for 7 1/2 years**
- **Employed as a teacher of English conversation**

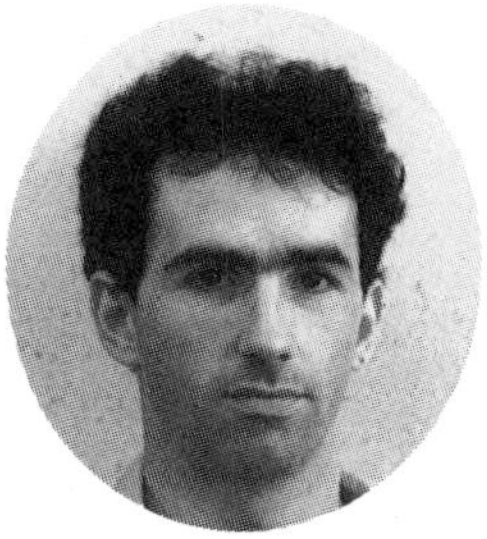

"*I used to suffer asthma attacks lasting four to five hours*"

At the age of 15 I moved with my family from Great Britain to New Zealand. Seven and half years ago I came to Japan because this land has always fascinated me. In fact I majored in Japanese language at my college in New Zealand, and presently teach English to the Japanese.

Why did I turn to Kampo when I came to Japan? Because nothing else had cured my asthma. When I was about two or three years old, I often had asthma attacks. Then the attacks disappeared, so I thought I had been cured. However, when I was 18, the attacks returned. That is common among asthma sufferers. It is often said that one can never be cured of asthma.

When I had my attacks, I would suffer from constant wheezing, coughing, and uncomfortable mucus buildup. If you have never suffered an asthma attack, I don't think you can imagine how miserable it can be. At the very least, the attacks would last an hour. The maximum would be four to five hours of non-stop coughing. When I first came to Japan, I experienced these attacks at least once or twice a month, sometimes more often than that.

I went to an orthodox doctor and explained my asthmatic history. He gave me an antihistamine, which is frequently prescribed for asthmatics. Although it helped control the wheezing, it left me drowsy.

It is common knowledge that asthma attacks get worse when one lies down. If I had an attack during the night, I would have to stay awake until it passed. What with lack of sleep and my generally run-down physical condition, I became a total wreck.

With each attack, I found myself relying more and more on the antihistamine to get badly needed rest, but was making no progress toward a genuine recovery. I decided to try changing my diet, with some good results, but I was still not cured.

"*Then I heard that kampo could cure asthma*"

Three years ago, a friend who was studying Kampo told me it could help asthmatic conditions. I decided to give it a try and went to Kitasato University for an examination. The questionnaire they had me fill out was very detailed. It asked for such information as a history of other illnesses I might have had besides asthma, and frequency and condition of urination, changes in appetite, throat and mouth condition, and overall physical state.

This part of the examination is called Monshin (Mon=questioning, shin=examination). Next, the doctor began Fukushin (fuku=abdomen), an examination of my abdomen by palpation. I had always believed asthma to be a condition of the lungs. I was very surprised when the problem was found to be in my stomach. Not only did the doctors check my pulse, they also checked my heartbeat for strong and weak pulsation. This is called Myakushin (myaku=heartbeat).

After this lengthy examination, the doctors prescribed a Kampo formula called *Sho-saiko-to*. The herbs in this remedy are also good for inflammation of the bronchial passages, for colds, and for chronic abdominal conditions. (I learned how effective it was for colds when I was given that same remedy for a cold I caught after my treatment for asthma.)

I continued taking *Sho-saiko-to* for two weeks. When I ran out of it, I went back to Kitasato University for a refill.

On the second visit, the doctors again performed Fukushin and Myakushin. This time they prescribed a formula called *Sho-seiryu-to*. That, they told me, was good for such symptoms as inflamed bronchial passages, bronchial asthma, runny nose, and inflamed sinus tissues. I took *Sho-seiryu-to* for six months. The doctors advised me to continue the medication even after the attack abated. I followed their instructions carefully.

The medicine worked. Little by little, I found my attacks decreasing. When I did have an attack, it was much lighter than before, and of shorter duration. With the onset of each attack or when I felt one coming, I would take my *Sho-seiryu-to*.

I have found my condition markedly improved. Knock on wood—I have not had an attack since the autumn of last year.

I have been told that remedies such as this one, which use natural barks and grasses, are entirely safe. That is the basis of herbal medicine, and I think it is right.

I have become a Kampo enthusiast and so has my wife. When she was pregnant, her morning sickness was terrible. The doctors prescribed a remedy called *Sho-hange-ka-bukuryo-to*. She has been very healthy and has experienced no discomfort.

EXPLANATION OF THE KAMPO MEDICINES DESCRIBED IN CASE STUDY #1

SHO-SAIKO-TO

Kampo ingredients (numbers indicate dosage in grams):

- Chinese Thoroughwax; Bepleurum Chinese..7
- Pinellia Ternata..5
- Ginger..4
- Baical Skullcap; Scutellaria baicalensis..3
- Giant Jujube Tree..3
- Ginseng..3
- Chinese licorice..2

• Symptoms indicating use:

- Loss of appetite
- Fever

• Conditions most used for:

- Pneumonia
- Inflamed bronchial passage
- Influenza
- Inflammation of chest tissues
- Tuberculosis and related diseases
- Inflamed lymph gland
- Chronic abdominal condition
- Liver conditions
- Postpartum recuperation

SHO-SEIRYU-TO

Kampo ingredients (numbers indicate dosage in grams):

- Ephedra vulgaris..3
- Peony..3
- Dried Ginger..3
- Chinese licorice..3
- Blume sticks; Cinnamomum cassia..3
- Asaiasarum sieboldi..3
- Pinellia ternata..6

• Symptoms indicating use:

- Coughing
- Wheezing
- Sneezing
- Runny nose

• Conditions most used for:

- Bronchial asthma
- Inflamed bronchial passages
- Inflamed bronchial passages due to asthma
- Allergies—runny nose
- Pneumonia
- Inflamed chest tissues
- Arthritis
- Tuberculosis
- Nephrosis
- Acute stages of nephritis (chronic inflammation of the kidneys)

SHO-HANGE-KA-BUKURYO-TO

Kampo ingredients (numbers indicate dosage in grams):

- Pinellia ternata..6
- Dried ginger..5
- Poria cocos..5

• Symptoms indicating use:

- Nausea
- Dizziness
- Heart palpitations
- Vomiting of milk by infants

• Conditions most used for:

- Morning sickness
- Vomiting

Case Study #2: Peter Yates, Age 34
- **Born in England**
- **Has lived in Japan for 15 months**

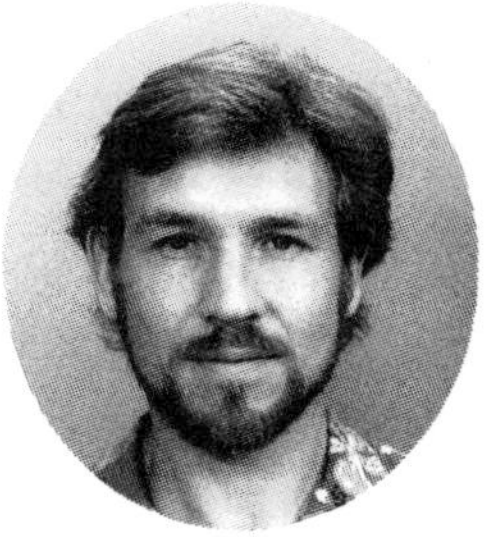

"Pain from over-exercising disappeared completely"
I enjoy traveling, and have visited the United States, Italy, Canada, Australia, Fiji, Singapore, and Taiwan. I had visited Japan once before, nine years ago.

For 20 years I have been on a fitness kick. In order to maintain good health, I have studied Oriental martial arts such as kung-fu, tae kwon do, and karate.

I discovered that besides martial arts, Japan has many other sources of knowledge for the health enthusiast. What I found most fascinating was Kampo. I was determined to study Kampo, and was very pleased to be admitted to the Asian Medicine Research Center in Mishima.

At first I had planned to study there for three months. Now I have arranged to extend my stay in Japan so I can study Kampo more thoroughly. Asian medicine, especially Kampo, uses complicated words and concepts. Since I don't know Japanese very well, and have difficulty reading Kanji (Chinese characters, used for formal printing in Japan), studying Kampo is very difficult for me. Because of my own experience, however, I can confidently recommend Kampo treatment to everyone.

I started having bad headaches about a year after coming to Japan. Also, my shoulders were stiff and my stomach felt distended and uneasy. At times I would seem quite well, and at other times would be anxious and irritable.

I was frustrated. My symptoms were clear but I didn't know their origin. I discussed my condition with a friend, who said it must be caused by "too much studying."

I recalled having had similar symptoms about three years earlier. At that time, I was introduced to a doctor who prescribed Kampo. I took *Dai-saiko-to*, which cured me in just one week.

"I felt at ease when the doctor examined me"
Naturally, I thought of Kampo immediately when this condition resurfaced. Best of all, I always feel at ease when the Kampo doctor examines me. How can I explain it? When I leave the doctor's office, I feel very relieved and as though I were already on the road to recovery.

Let me give an example. If you were to go to an orthodox medical doctor and tell him your head hurt, all he would do is examine your head. A Kampo doctor, however, will ask about changes in your appetite, urine and stool condition, and will check your tongue and even your heartbeat. He will then try to bring the entire body back to its normal working state. I think all medicine should be practiced this way.

When I went to the Kampo doctor with my problem, he prescribed *Dai-saiko-to* as the previous doctor had done. But I was also delighted to hear that I would not have to brew a tea of Kampo herbs. Instead, the medicine now came in tablet form which was much easier to take.

I took the tablets three times daily before meals. After two or three weeks, I had recovered completely and regained ample energy to continue my martial arts exercises.

"*Backaches almost cost me my job*"

One day as I was practicing martial arts, I felt a sharp pain that ran from my lower back down through my leg. I had received the same injury once before during karate practice. Since I am a karate instructor, I was quite worried. If I didn't do something quickly, I could lose my job.

I explained to the doctor that, if possible, I would like to cure the condition with Kampo. The doctor gave me a series of careful examinations and then prescribed *Sokkei-kakketsu-to*. In about a week, the pain disappeared.

Before I started taking this medication, I had experienced severe pain both before and after my workouts. I was amazed at how little time was required for me to feel almost complete relief with Kampo.

There are people who claim that Kampo is a slow cure. In my case, however, I find this to be untrue. Kampo won't cure you in the same way orthodox medicine does, for instance by alleviating a headache in one hour. Kampo rather finds *Sho* (basic malfunction) in each individual and prescribes whatever fits that individual's physical condition.

The reason I choose Kampo is because of its long history of success and its refinement through the ages. It has been used and proven effective for many, many generations.

EXPLANATION OF THE KAMPO MEDICINES DESCRIBED IN CASE STUDY #2

DAI-SAIKO-TO

Kampo Ingredients (numbers indicate dosage in grams):
- Bupleuri Radix. .6
- Pinelliae Tuber. .4
- Scutellariae Radix. .3
- Zizyphi Fructus. .3
- Aurantii Fructus Immaturus. .2
- Zingiberis Rhizoma. .1
- Rhei Rhizoma. .1

• Symptoms indicating use:
- Constipation
- Discomfort and distention of upper abdomen
- Tinnitus
- Stiff shoulders

• Conditions most used for:
- Gall stones
- Cholecystitis
- Jaundice
- Liver function disorders
- Hypertension
- Cerebral anemia
- Urticaria
- Gastric hyperacidity
- Acute gastoenteric catarrh
- Nausea
- Vomiting
- Loss of appetite
- Hemorrhoids
- Diabetes
- Neurosis
- Insomnia

SOKEI-KAKKETSU-TO

Kampo Ingredients (numbers indicate dosage in grams):
- Paeoniae Radix. .2.5
- Rehmanniae Radix. .2
- Cnidii Rhizoma. .2
- Atractylodis Lancea Rhizoma. .2
- Angelicae Radix. .2
- Persicae Semen. .2
- Hoelen. .2
- Achyranthis Radix. .1.5
- Aurantii Nobilis Pericarpium. .1.5
- Sinomeni Caulis et Rhizoma. .1.5
- Ledebouriellae Radix. .1.5
- Gentianae Scabrae Radix. .1.5
- Glycyrrhizae Radix. .1
- Angelicae Dahuricae Radix. .1
- Zingiberis Rhizoma. .0.5
- Clemantidis Radix. .1.5
- Notopterygii Rhizoma. .1.5

• Symptoms indicating use:
- Muscle, joint and nerve pain from lower back down to legs

• Conditions most used for:
- Joint pain
- Neuralgia
- Muscle pain

Case Study #3: Tom Walker, Age 42
- **Born in North Carolina, U.S.A.**
- **Has lived in Japan for 17 years**
- **Teaches English conversation**

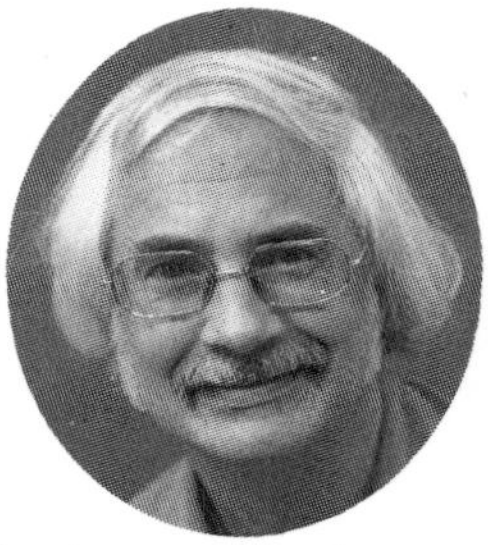

"*My Heart Would Palpitate For No Reason*"

I was in the U.S. Navy during the Vietnam War. I have admired Japan ever since we stopped in that country on our way to Vietnam. After my discharge from the Navy, I returned to the United States but soon came back to Japan. I've been here 17 years now and am presently teaching at an English Conversation School in Yotsuya, Tokyo.

My students are serious about their studies and I enjoy my work very much. One thing, however, was troubling me. From time to time I would experience severe heart palpitations. After they became worse, I quit smoking. Even then the chest pains did not stop, so a month later I went to Shibuya to see a doctor. He took blood tests, heart x-rays, and heart pulsation tests, but found nothing physically wrong with me.

I continued to experience severe chest pains, but without a diagnosis there could be no help. In fact, being told there was nothing wrong left me feeling afraid and insecure. When I told the doctor I had quit smoking, he advised me to stop drinking coffee as well. I really enjoy both those things and found it very hard to do without them. Finally I did quit drinking coffee in the hope that this second step might cure me at last. Another month passed without any change. Those alarming chest pains would not go away. When I slept, the pains were even worse.

I went back to the doctor and was given some more examinations. Again they found nothing physically wrong with me except that my blood pressure was a little low.

I am 175 cm (5 ft 9 in) tall and weigh 71.5 kg (159 lbs). I asked the doctor if my problem might be due to overweight. He said I was in good physical condition and didn't need to worry. When I told him my chest pains became worse at night, he prescribed tranquilizers. In spite of all the trouble I went through to get the prescription, it did nothing for me. There were many nights when I couldn't sleep at all, and I felt increasingly worse.

I worried that the lack of sleep might affect my work. Recalling that when I was younger I used to have a few drinks in order to sleep better, I started drinking alcohol before going to bed. Even that did nothing to ease the chest pains. I could both feel and hear my heart beating heavily, and still could not get a good night's rest.

"*The Mysterious Odor of Brewed Medicine*"

It was at this time that I met a friend who was studying Kampo. When I told him about my condition, he suggested that I try Kampo and explained how it works.

The Kampo doctor took note of my symptoms, and then examined my heartbeat, tongue, and abdomen. I remember wondering why the doctor checked my tongue when it was my heart that was giving me trouble.

After this thorough examination, he prescribed *Saiko-ka-ryukotsu-borei-to*. The medication looked like grass and white powder. I had always thought medicine came in the form of capsules and tablets and did not see how I could put this into my mouth.

The doctor explained that I was to brew the medicine and drink its broth. I went home and immediately tried it. The smell it produced was amazing. My entire kitchen was filled with the scent—strong, but not unpleasant. The taste was like nothing I had ever tried before, but it wasn't bad. At first it seemed odd to be making my own medicine, but soon I began to enjoy the task.

"*Took Three Times More Than I Should Have*"

I had fun making my brew, but after about five days my two-week supply of medicine was gone. That seemed strange, so I called the doctor. He told me I had made a mistake and was taking a triple dosage every day!

Imagine what would have happened if I had overdosed on tranquilizers. With this natural medicine, however, no matter how much I took, there were no side-effects. The doctor explained that that was an important difference between Kampo and modern orthodox medicine.

"Five days have passed," he said, "and you have not experienced any side-effects. I doubt if you will suffer any now. Side-effects from Kampo would appear only if the medication did not agree with your *sho* (condition)."

At first I was doubtful about Kampo, but within two weeks my heart palpitations had disappeared. I continued taking the medication for a while longer and then stopped. From that time on, I have not experienced any chest pains.

I do not know the theories or the composition of Kampo. After experiencing its effectiveness, however, and the thorough examinations and explanations of the doctors, I really believe in it. When I was experiencing the pains, I kept going around in the same circle: chest pains, insomnia, anger, irritability, depression. Sometimes I even felt like dying. With Kampo, I was able to break that cycle. I really feel it is superior to orthodox medicine and I tell that to everyone I meet.

EXPLANATION OF THE KAMPO MEDICINES DESCRIBED IN CASE STUDY #3

SAIKO-KA-RYUKOTSU-BOREI-TO

Kampo Ingredients (numbers indicate dosage in grams):

- Bupleuri Radix..5
- Pinelliae Tuber..4
- Cinnamomi Cortex..3
- Hoelen..3
- Scutellariae Radix..2.5
- Zizyphi Fructus..2.5
- Ginseng Radix..2.5
- Ostreae Testa..2.5
- Fossilia Ossis Mastodi..2.5
- Zingiberis Rhizoma..1

- Symptoms indicating use:
  - Tachycardia
  - Insomnia
  - Irritability
- Conditions most used for:
  - Hypertension
  - Arteriosclerosis
  - Chronic kidney diseases
  - Neurasthenia
  - Neurotic tachycardia
  - Epilepsy
  - Hysteria
  - Children's night crying
  - Impotence

"A wise person considers health to be the greatest of human blessings."
—Hippocrates of Cos

CHAPTER 5

THE FUTURE OF KAMPO MEDICINE

One hundred years ago Japan emerged from its long period of seclusion and quickly developed into a new society based on western ideas and science. The government gave orders that western medicine was to be practiced nationally. As a result, the number of Kampo practitioners dropped sharply and the medieval art of Kampo was almost lost.

In recent years, some of the doctors who had continued to practice traditional medicine became disgruntled with the government's discriminatory policies and issued a challenge to see whether diabetes could be cured more effectively by eastern or western-style medicine. Kampo proved to be the better cure, but the government refused to change its policies. Western medicine remained in vogue with full official sanction.

Establishing Kampo's validity is an immediate priority and research is underway for the systematic collection of data. In 1976, a number of Kampo medications were finally approved by the Japanese government.

In November 1982, 4290 of the physicians in Japan responding to a questionnaire by the *Nikkei Medical Journal* acknowledged that they gave Kampo prescriptions. Recently, a number of centers have been created for research into Kampo. Among these are the Japan Kampo Research Center, the Kitasato Research Center, and centers at Kinki University and Toyama Medical University. Research and testing is also being carried out in the research and development divisions of pharmaceutical manufacturers, such as Tsumura & Co. in Japan, and in many national and public hospital facilities, as well as university-owned hospitals.

Because so many clinical research centers have been created and so much research on Kampo has been reported in the past ten years, Kampo is now being discussed at many medical conferences. For instance, the Japan Dermatology Association, the Japan Gynecology Association, the Japan Digestive System and Disease Association, the Japan Pharmaceutical Association and the International Internal Medicine Association have all made reports on Kampo usage. Information and awareness of Kampo is also increasing the number of courses they offer.

Kampo medicine and allopathic medicine have very different backgrounds. Yet they exist side-by-side and often both are used by clinical physicians in Japan today.

Despite their difference, they have the same objective: to cure the sick. Each, too, has special curative abilities. If practitioners were to use the best of both fields, the effectiveness of each in curing illness would be greatly enhanced.

PART THREE

Examination and Treatment in Kampo

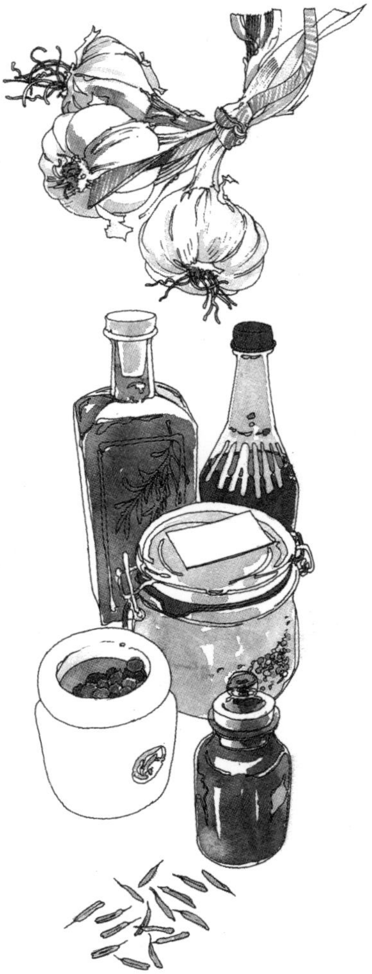

"An open mind is the moral essence of medicine."

—Dr. Taro Takemi, M.D.
Pres., World Medical Assn.

CHAPTER 1

CANCER

What is Cancer?

Most people are not aware that at any time normal cells can suddenly become cancerous, even when a person is apparently in the "best of health." Most of the time, however, a natural resistance—or immune response capacity—destroys these cancerous tumors at a very early stage of development.

Even when a certain minimal amount of disease causing agents enter the body, illness may not occur if at the same time the body's strength, immunity and other self-defensive systems are able to protect the body. However, once the body lapses into a weakened condition and self-defensive capability is no longer effective, what were up until now normal cells can suddenly change. These changed cells can increase and grow and go on to invade healthy parts of the body. These cancer cells then move throughout the body through the blood and/or lymph systems, multiplying and eventually causing death.

The Effect of Kampo on Cancer

Western anticancer drugs work because they have DNA synthesis inhibiting properties. These prevent cancer cells from dividing and thus multiplying, by destroying the DNA which composes the nucleus of the cancer cells. Although it is true that cancer cells are killed by these drugs, the DNA of normal cells is also destroyed, thereby dealing a body blow to healthy organs essential to the maintenance of life. In addition there is a reduction in the amount of white blood cells, bacteria and other foreign substances. These are normally found in the lymph nodes, spleen, bone marrow, etc. Also, with cancer therapy there is a loss of appetite, loss of hair and other side effects which cause a further weakening of the body, and tragically hurry the patient further along the road to death.

In cases where there is surgical removal of advanced cancer, this drastic procedure adversely affects the various functions of the internal organs and further weakens the body. When this is combined with post-surgical treatment with anticancer drugs, the side effects only speed up the weakening of the body's strength– including its immune response capability.

For the reasons mentioned here, it is important to first nourish and strengthen the cancer patients' over-all condition, including the immune system, in order to heighten their resistance.

The growing use of Kampo treatments simultaneously with western drugs, surgery and other treatment prevents side effects from occurring. Kampo treatment not only regulates the immune, hormone and nervous systems and thereby strengthens the body's own natural healing power, but also prevents many of the harmful side effects which accompany the administration of DNA synthesis inhibiting drugs, such as: reduction of white blood cells, loss of appetite, and lowering of the function of the reticulo-endothelial system. This fact was established from the point of view of western medicine. In this respect the Japan Medical Association made an important step in the recognition of the usefulness of Kampo medicine.

Treatment with Kampo

Previously Kampo prescriptions were believed to attack the cancer indirectly by strengthening the body, increasing the appetite, increasing resistance to disease and, at the same time, reducing the side effects of anticancer drugs.

However, in 1986 it was reported at the Japan Medical Association that certain types of Kampo medicines do act directly on the cancer. The medications are toxic to cancerous cells without doing any harm to the healthy cells. This is considered a medical breakthrough in terms of western medicine.

In the actual case studies that follow, Kampo prescriptions were used to prevent the side effects caused by the use of chemotherapy and immunotherapy on post-surgical patients. The data from 42 universities throughout Japan was collected by Professor Nabetani of Japan's Kyorin University surgery department with the participation of Dr. Monma (representing Professor Tajima) of Dokkyo University's Surgical Department.

The majority of the patients in the clinical experiments had resections done on esophagus cancer, stomach cancer, colon cancer, etc. These patients were split into two groups: The "A" group received chemotherapy and immunotherapy, and were administered 25 g of the Kampo prescription Juzen-Taiho-To three times per day (a total of 75 g/day), after meals, for 12 weeks. The "B" group was under the same conditions as the "A" group, except they did not receive Juzen-Taiho-To.

The results are as follows:

1) Effect on subjective symptoms (increase of appetite, reduction of general fatigue, etc.):
    A group: over 90% effective
    B group: 60—70% effective

2) Effect on preventing side effects of chemotherapy and immunotherapy (skin eruptions, pigmentation and other skin complaints, stomatitis, and other similar symptoms):
   A group: 22—40% had symptoms
   B group: 30—60% had symptoms
3) Effect on body weight (see diagram 1):

Many medical organizations, including top-class university hospitals in Japan, have now included Kampo therapy as a permanent part of the treatment in cancer. They have reported that Juzen-Taiho-To prevents the reduction in the number of white blood cells as a result of radiotherapy and that it may also reduce the danger of infection due to a loss of white blood cells.

Actual Examples of Treatment

To prevent side effects of anticancer drugs and immunotherapy and to prevent the loss of body strength due to the cancer itself and/or surgery.

JUZEN-TAIHO-TO: This is administered to patients in various weakened conditions, such as post-illness, post-surgery and chronic illnesses. The general symptoms that it can alleviate are extreme fatigue, pale complexion, loss of appetite, dry or scaly skin, night sweat, and dryness of the mouth. It is administered to hospital inpatients.

HOCHU-EKKI-TO: This is administered to patients with slightly more strength and stamina than the patients to whom the above prescription (Juzen-Taiho-To) is administered. This is used for chronic illness, anemia, and post-surgical conditions where there is continuous fatigue, loss of appetite, coughing, low grade fever, night sweat, palpitations, anxiety, etc. It is appropriate for hospital out-patients.

	Weight pre-surgery (1 m 16s)	Weight 1 month after surgery	Weight 5 mos. after surgery	Net gain or loss
JUZEN-TAIHO-TO Group (average)	109.6	105.6	112.4	+2.8
Control Group (average)	104.5	95.9	101.8	−3.7

Diagram 1 Effect on body weight

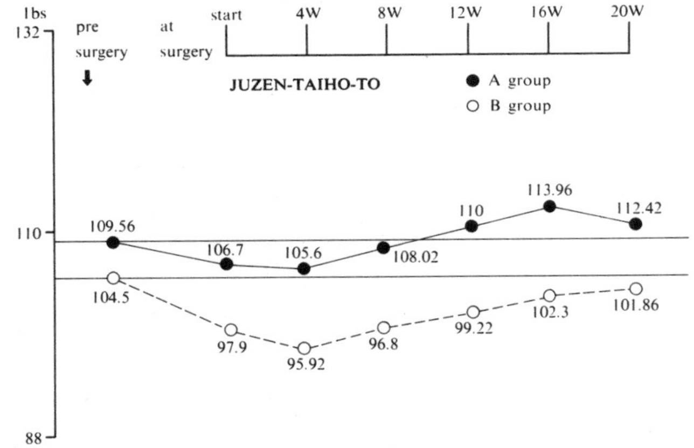

Diagram 2 Number of white blood cells

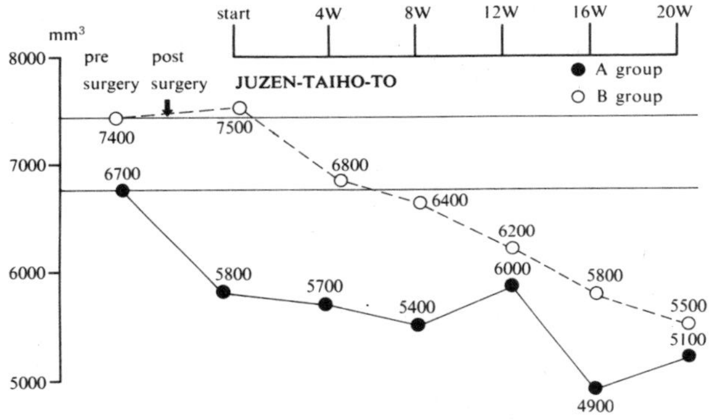

Diagram 3 Number of lymph cells

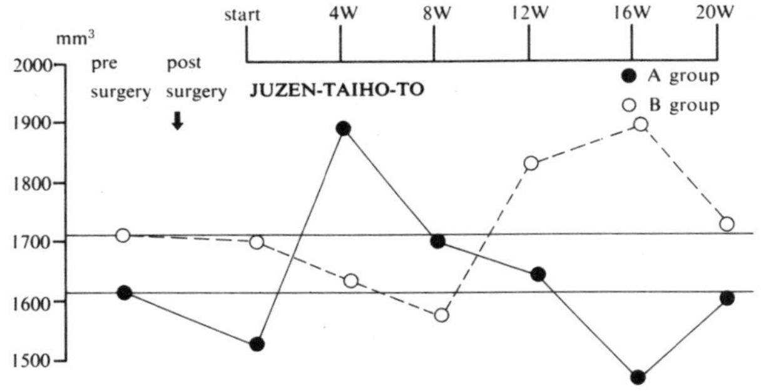

Number of white blood cells and number of lymph cells

Although there was a reduction in the number of white blood cells in B group there was very little reduction in A group. JUZEN-TAIHO-TO prevented a reduction in the amount of white blood cells, A group also showed a slight increase in the amount of lymph cells as compared with B group. (Diagrams 2 and 3)

CHAPTER 2

LIVER DISEASES

The liver is the largest organ in the body and is responsible for the essential functions of storing, detoxifying, disassimilation and excretion of nutritive substances. The liver plays a central role in the life of the organism. There are many types of liver diseases: acute hepatitis, cirrhosis of the liver, portal hypertension, liver cancer and fatty liver are a few. Hepatitis is the most prevalent. The causes of acute hepatitis include virus attack, drugs, alcohol and post-surgical trauma. Four viruses attack the liver: A type, B type non-A, and non-B type.

About 10 to 20% of acute hepatitis cases become chronic. "Chronic hepatitis" occurs when there is acute hepatitis with the liver function failing to normalize after 6 months. It is known that about 10% of all chronic hepatitis ends in cirrhosis of the liver. This may then go on to become liver cancer. Therefore, the central emphasis of modern treatment is to prevent hepatitis from becoming chronic. Histologically speaking, the liver cells become fibrous along with inflammation. Thirty percent of chronic hepatitis is B-type virus, and it is assumed that the rest are caused from continuous infection from a non-A and non-B type virus. Since the non-A and non-B type viruses have not yet been isolated, this is an extremely difficult problem to treat.

The Effect of Kampo on Liver Function Disorders

Even in modern medicine, there is no fixed method of treatment for chronic hepatitis. Recently, antiviral drugs and immuno-regulating drugs have been used. So far, however, these drugs have not been proven effective. In addition to these drugs, therefore, physicians strongly recommend therapy and rest.

There are many Kampo medicines used for liver function disorders, but the most important and frequently used are prescriptions which contain the crude drug bupleurum (umbelliferae, the radix of bupleurum falcatum and other similar varieties). It is, however, important to use formulas which suit each individual patient.

Research on the effects of Kampo medicines on liver disorders is advancing and the following properties have been scientifically proven: they protect the membrane of the liver cells, strengthen reproduction of liver cells, increase liver blood flow, and also have a valuable immuno-regulating effect.

Treatment with Kampo

In most cases, after taking Kampo medicine for 2 to 4 weeks, the subjective symptoms of loss of appetite, fatigue, etc., are the first to improve, followed by improvement in liver function based on test results (GOT, GPT, etc.). Although there is a common tendency for chronic hepatitis to worsen and recur, under most treatment, cases stabilize. As hepatitis is a difficult illness to treat, patients should always be under the care and treatment of a doctor and have monthly clinical tests.

Actual Examples of Treatment

DAI-SAIKO-TO: Used when patient is relatively energetic and examination reveals pain and distention under both sides of the ribs on the abdomen (hypochondrium) and discomfort when pressed. Other symptoms include constipation and stiff shoulders.

SHO-SAIKO-TO: For patients with average energy and strength, discomfort and distention under the right side of the ribs on the upper part of the abdomen, loss of appetite, accompanied by fatigue and/or a white coating on the tongue and/or a bitter taste and discomfort in the mouth.

SAIKO-KEISHI-TO: For patients with slightly weak constitution, discomfort and pain under the right side of the ribs on the upper abdomen, tense abdominus rectus, tendency to perspire and have headrushes and stiff shoulders.

HOCHU-EKKI-TO: For those in a very weak condition with loss of appetite and severe fatigue.

KEISHI-BUKURYO-GAN: To be used with those who experience pain when pressure is applied to the lower abdomen; red-black tongue/lips, and small blood vessel easily seen in the face and chest area or red spots on the palms of the hands. This may be used along with the above prescriptions.

CHAPTER 3

CHRONIC GASTRITIS

One of the most common problems for contemporary man is overeating. This is a serious health problem which can wreak havoc with the digestive system and may eventually lead to acute gastritis leading to chronic gastritis.

The symptoms of acute gastritis are discomfort, a distended feeling in the abdomen, stomach pain, nausea, and loss of appetite. This illness is most often brought on by the consumption of difficult to digest, tainted, or cold food. Symptoms are usually alleviated after two or three days. If overeating and snacking while watching TV become habitual, continuous symptoms such as pain, discomfort, pressure, and heaviness in the epigastrium, heartburn, acidic belching, vomiting, and loss of appetite can occur. The most common form of gastritis is atrophic gastritis, in which the mucous membrane of the stomach becomes atrophic with age. Advanced symptoms include continuous inflammation of the stomach mucous membrane, atrophy of the gastric glands and thickening of the folds above the mucous membrane. These symptoms are caused by external factors such as food, alcohol, tobacco and irritating substances. Internal factors, such as stress and emotional disturbance, compound the problem.

The Effect of Kampo on Chronic Gastritis

Modern medicine treats only the symptoms of patients with chronic gastritis. In Kampo medicine, however, illness is seen from a holistic point of view. Emphasis is put on improving the natural healing power of the body and restoring the body's balance. Kampo treatment of chronic gastritis includes improving blood circulation and aiding the body's own natural healing capabilities. Kampo helps calm excited mental states, relieves tiredness and fatigue, and where called for, increases the appetite, aiding in a healthy increase of weight.

People prone to chronic gastritis usually have a relatively weak constitution. Kampo treatments correct this by improving the metabolism and strengthening the body.

Actual Examples of Treatment

ANCHU-SAN: Used for those in a relatively weak condition, in whom the gastritis has become chronic, together with stomach pain and heartburn.

HANGE-SHASHIN-TO: Used for those who have an average constitution, in whom the epigastrium feels blocked, with borborygmus (belly rumbles), nausea, vomiting, and diarrhea.

RIKKUNSHI-TO: Used for those with a relatively weak constitution who have a loss of strength, loss of appetite, general fatigue, discomfort in the epigastrium, and who tend to have cold extremities. (Often used for elderly people.)

SHIGYAKU-SAN: Used for those with above average constitution, strong discomfort in the chest, anxiety, insomnia, depression and other emotional disturbances.

CHAPTER 4

HYPERTENSION (High Blood Pressure)

According to the World Health Organization hypertension is a condition in which the systolic blood pressure is about 160 mmHG and the diastolic blood pressure is above 95 mmHG.

There are many factors which cause the blood pressure to rise. They include: nervous factors such as stress; loss of elasticity of the walls of the blood vessels and reduction of the internal diameter of blood vessels due to aging; overconsumption of sodium (table salt); and illnesses of the kidneys and adrenals. A great number of hypertension cases, however, have no clear causes and are referred to as essential hypertension.

The Effect of Kampo on Hypertension

The hypotensive action of Kampo medicines is generally mild compared with the usual western medicine. Since hypertension occurs due to an upset in the blood pressure regulating structure, it is mainly thought of as a constitutional illness. Kampo treatment addresses the entire constitution. It stabilizes the central nervous system (which is thought of as being the trigger of hypertension), improves high blood fat and blood mucosity (which are the cause of thrombosis and the transformation of red blood cells), regulates electrolytes such as sodium, tranquilizes thereby reducing stress, brings about an overall balance in the organs, relieving headaches, anxiety, stiff shoulders, vertigo, and most important, lowers blood pressure.

When Kampo medicines are administered to hypertensive patients in the early stages of treatment, the symptoms of discomfort such as stiff shoulders, headaches, headrushes, and anxiety frequently disappear immediately. Then the blood pressure gradually starts to drop. Finally, Kampo works a complete cure. Even if the Kampo medicine is not taken for some time, the blood pressure remains low. There is seldom, if ever, a relapse.

Treatment with Kampo

Kampo is most appropriate for treating hypertension where the systolic pressure is between 160 and 180 and the diasystolic between 95 and 100. It may also be used to treat cases that are in the gray zone between hypertension and normal blood pressure.

However, when a malignant type of hypertension such as renal hypertension exists, or when the blood pressure is extremely high, or if the symptoms do not respond to treatment, then it is important that stronger hypertensives be administered by a doctor.

Actual Examples of Treatment

When the patient's diastolic pressure is high:
SHICHIMOTSU-KOKA-TO: For average patients.

When the patient experiences headaches (especially early in the morning), stiff shoulders, etc.:
CHOTO-SAN: For average patients.

When the patient experiences headrushes and anxiety:
OREN-GEDOKU-TO: For average patients.
SAN'O-SHASHIN-TO: For average patients with constipation.
SAIKO-KA-RYUKOTSU-BOREI-TO: For above average patients with strong constitutions.

CHAPTER 5

HYPERLIPIDISM AND ARTERIOSCLEROSIS

Hyperlipidism is a condition where there is an increase of triglycerides in the blood with cloudy blood serum. The causes range from over-consumption of fatty foods, heredity, and secondary symptoms from illness to irregularities in the body's metabolism.

Arteriosclerosis occurs when the arteries lose their elasticity, and become hard, and the internal diameter narrows. There are three types: senile arteriosclerosis; "gruel" type sclerosis; and arteriosclerosis. The causes differ depending upon the type, but it is thought that they all result from a combination of aging, hereditary factors, hypertension or hyperlipidism. Other factors that contribute to arteriosclerosis include diabetes, obesity, stress, and cigarette smoking.

The Effect of Kampo on Hyperlipidism and Arteriosclerosis

A certain amount of effectiveness is gained through the use of western drugs to treat hyperlipidism and arteriosclerosis. Kampo is also effective in treating arteriosclerosis-related illnesses and safer to use.

Among the crude drugs, such as coptidis, bupleurum, ginseng, etc., which comprise Kampo formulas, there are those which lower blood lipid levels and increase the amount of HD cholesterol—lessening the danger of hardening of the arteries. Kampo prevents and alleviates hyperlipidism and arteriosclerosis.

Also, as vascular dilators are successfully used in the treatment of arteriosclerosis, their counterparts such as cinnamon, uncaria, ginseng and angelica acutiloba are now being used to dilate the peripheral blood vessels.

There are also illnesses which occur due to arteriosclerosis, such as "blood insufficiency" type illnesses. These occur when the internal diameter of the blood vessels becomes narrow, preventing enough oxygen and nourishment to reach the extremities. If this occurs in the aorta, angina pectoris or myocardial infarction may be the result. If it occurs in the brain, cerebral thrombosis, cerebral embolism or temporary cerebral blood insufficiency attacks may occur. In modern medical treatment of these illnesses, antiplatelet therapy is used. However, this prevents coagulation of the platelets in the blood, and hemorrhaging becomes the risk. Thrombosis-dissolving agents such as Urokinase-(UK) are also frequently used.

Among the crude drugs used in Kampo formulas, there are some which supress cohesion of blood platelets, i.e. they speed up the dissolution of those that have already hardened (thrombus). Cinnamon, peach kernels and giant peony root are some examples. However, as their effect is not as strong as western drugs, it is believed they are most useful in prevention rather than in the cure of dangerous conditions.

Treatment with Kampo

As mentioned previously, Kampo medicines, due to the various properties of their crude drugs, regulate the lipid tissue in the blood (metabolism), regulate the blood coagulation system and remove stress, and are therefore useful in treating arteriosclerosis as well as preventing a variety of blood disorders.

Actual Examples of Treatment

When there is cerebral thrombosis:

CHOTO-SAN: For the early stages when symptoms include headaches. There may also be stiff shoulders and forgetfulness.

SAN'O-SHASHIN-TO: For patients with relatively strong constitutions. Symptoms include anxiety, headrushes, and constipation.

OREN-GEDOKU-TO: Used for the same symptoms above, except there is no constipation.

SAIKO-KA-RYUKOTSU-BOREI-TO: For patients with strong constitutions with symptoms of anxiety, insomnia, other nervous symptoms, and palpitations.

When there is hardening of the aorta:

OBOI-TO: For relatively weak patients showing shortness of breath, palpitations, pressure in the chest, and a blocked feeling in the epigastrium.

When there is hardening of the arteries of the lower extremities:

HACHIMI-JIO-GAN: For cases with severe fatigue, nocturia (urinating at night), lower back pain. Also used when there is hardening of the kidneys.

CHAPTER 6

APOPLEXY (Stroke)

After a sudden disturbance of the brain's blood circulation, problems with consciousness, speech, and movement can appear. These disturbances in circulation are divided into two major categories. The first occurs when the brain's blood vessels become blocked (cerebral thrombosis) and the second occurs when the brain's blood vessels burst (cerebral hemorrhage).

The Effect of Kampo on Apoplexy

Although western medicine and/or surgery are necessary directly after an attack of apoplexy, once the acute stage is over and the patient's condition has settled and rehabilitation has begun, Kampo is useful in the recovery of strength. It reduces danger of post-attack symptoms such as numbness, paralysis of the extremities, and other motor impediments and nerve paralysis.

Apoplexy does not usually occur suddenly without warning. Often there are warning signs, such as continuous high blood pressure preceding the attack. Kampo administered when these signs appear can prevent an attack from occurring.

Treatment with Kampo

Kampo can treat paralysis as well as speed recovery. The herbal mixtures are administered according to each patient's illness and symptoms, whether they are hypertension, hyperlipidism, heart disease, or diabetes. Patients are also advised to use modern drugs along with Kampo and to remove stress that causes attacks.

Kampo crude drugs such as San'o-Shashin-To and Oren-Gedoku-To, taken when thrombosis threatens, can prevent the coagulation of blood and blockage.

Actual Example of Treatment

In cases where there is paralysis, motor impediments, and numbness:

ZOKUMEI-TO: Used for patients with average constitution.

SHIMBU-TO: Used for weak patients.

KEISHI-KA-JUTSUBU-TO: For relatively weak patients who feel cold and perspire easily.

For cases of mental disturbances with anxiety, short temper, insomnia:

SAIKO-KA-RYUKOTSU-BOREI-TO: For patients with strong constitution. May also be used for arteriosclerosis.

To prevent attacks when there is a tendency toward arteriosclerosis or hyperlipidism:

OREN-GEDOKU-TO: For average patients, with mental and nervous symptoms.

SAN'O-SHASHIN-TO: For patients with strong constitutions, having headrushes and constipation.

CHAPTER 7

HEART DISEASES

There are various types of heart disease, categorized by the damaged part of the heart and the cause of the damage. Here is a simple classification of various heart diseases:

Classification according to location:

1) Heart blood vessels (aorta): Angina pectoris, myocardial infarction.
   The main cause is a hardening of the aorta which can result in a lack of oxygen and nourishment reaching the heart. When the aorta temporarily closes and the heart muscle becomes short of oxygen, there is a tightening pain in the chest. This is called "angina pectoris". This pain usually abates within a few minutes. If the aorta becomes totally blocked and causes the death of heart muscle cells, it is called "myocardial infarction."
2) Heart internal membrane: valvular heart disease.
   This is a disturbance of the four valves which aid in the pumping action of the heart, and results when they fail to open and close as they should. It can be caused by a congenital condition, by bacterial infection, or an attack of rheumatism.

Classification according to causes:

1) Hereditary
   Distortion of the heart which may occur during the first three months of pregnancy if the mother contracts rubella.
2) Rheumatism
   Valvular problems due to an attack of rheumatic fever.
3) Bacterial
   Heart muscle inflammation, heart membrane malformation.
4) Other

The Effect of Kampo on Heart Disease

Although one must proceed with extreme caution and care when treating such life-threatening diseases such as myocardial infarction, this does not preclude the use of Kampo medicine.

Kampo is the best choice when the patient is able to carry on a normal, existence. Kampo is especially useful if the patient is already receiving treatment from a doctor and there is no immediate danger to life. For example, Kampo will help in cases of angina, irregular pulse, and acute left ventricle insufficiency. However, Kampo is not appropriate for acute stages of heart disease.

If Kampo therapy is skillfully used along with western medicine, symptoms such as chest pain, shortness of breath and palpitations can be effectively reduced.

Treatment with Kampo

Treatment with Kampo is appropriate for the non-acute angina stage. In cases of chronic but less serious myocardial infarction, Kampo may be used to prevent recurring symptoms after a severe attack.

1) Light angina pectoris.
   Kampo may be used along with other medicines such as ß blocker, aorta dilators and calcium antagonizing drugs to reduce the frequency and strength of attacks.
2) Myocardial infarction.
   Kampo is often effective for reducing the frequency of attacks and also aids in the rehabilitation process that is necessary after a serious attack by increasing the blood flow through the aorta.
3) Light cardiac insufficiency.
   Kampo may help ease the symptoms of chest pain, shortness of breath and palpitations if used along with digitalis, heart tonics, diuretics, and other heart drugs.

Actual Examples of Treatment

Angina, after light myocardial infarction attack.

For patients with an average constitution:
KARO-GAIHAKU-HAKUSHU-TO: For those who experience pain that spreads from the ribs and heart area to the back.

For patients with a weakened constitution:
MOKU-BOI-TO: For cases with a blocked feeling in the epigastrium, respiratory difficulties, palpitations, and the possibility of edema.

TOKI-TO: For those with a cold constitution, pale complexion, and pain that spreads from the chest to the back.

For patients with irregular pulse:
SHA-KANZO-TO: For patients in a weakened condition with scaly dry skin, who tire easily, and experience hotness of hands and feet.

CHAPTER 8

AUTONOMIC NERVOUS SYSTEM

Fortunately, the human body is miraculously automatic. Even if subjected to mental and physical stress, a mechanism protects us from harm. When this mechanism, the autonomic nervous system, is disturbed and does not function properly, we become ill.

There are two types of disturbances: first, where the mental and physical balance is upset by being subjected to too much stress, and the second, where the mind and body are already so weak that only a small amount of stress is enough to cause a severe disturbance or illness.

The symptoms of this second condition are general fatigue, vertigo, headaches, a heavy feeling in the head, palpitation, stomach and intestinal symptoms, irregular perspiration, hotness, headrushes, cold hands and feet, insomnia and many others.

The Effect of Kampo on Disturbances of the Autonomic Nervous System

One of Kampo's unique features is that it does not have the side effect of depressing the central nervous system (sleepiness, loss of energy, faintness) that psychotropics have. It also does not cause drug-related liver complaints or drug dependency.

The effect of Kampo on nervous symptoms such as anxiety, tension, and depression are mild compared with western psychotropics, but if the appropriate Kampo prescription is administered, good results and often a complete cure can be expected. In most cases, improvement can be seen within a month and it is not necessary to continue treatment longer than six months.

Treatment with Kampo

Although there are presently many methods to treat disturbances of the autonomic nervous system, a good relationship between the therapist or doctor and the patient is indispensable for successful treatment.

Although many cases are cured with standard western treatment, relapses often occur when drug therapy is discontinued. These cases are the most difficult to treat. Kampo, however, can give hope to many of these patients. Even the most difficult cases have a good chance of recovery using a combination of Kampo with psychotropics.

Actual Examples of Treatment

In cases where there is hotness in the upper half of the body and coldness in the legs:
KAMI-SHOYO-SAN: For women with weak constitutions.

When vertigo and faintness are experienced.
RYO-KYO-JUTSU-KAN-TO: For relatively weak patients.

If symptoms include palpitations, anxiety and insomnia:
SAIKO-KA-RYUKOTSU-BOREI-TO: For relatively strong patients.

Throat feels blocked, always complains of discomfort.
HANGE-KOBOKU-TO: For average strength patients.

If the patient is excited, anxious, and has a short temper.
YOKU-KAN-SAN-KA-CHIMPI-HANGE: For relatively weak patients.

CHAPTER 9

OBESITY

Obesity is a problem in highly developed countries where food is abundant. It rarely exists where there is a shortage of food.

There are many cases of obesity in America, even many cases of severe obesity. The main contributing factor is overconsumption of calories and especially the consumption of high fat foods. In addition, there is usually a complete lack of exercise. Under these conditions, calories are stored by the body as fat.

Although there are certain cases which are caused through irregularities in the internal secretion system (hormones), most are caused through overeating. The primary type of obesity is the inherited constitution of obese parents, and the secondary type is the simple result of overeating.

One problem is that obesity is not seen as an illness. Yet, when compared with a person of normal weight, obese people tend to be much more susceptible to a variety of diseases. It is common knowledge among doctors that many obese-people suffer from diabetes, hypertension, hyperlipidism, arteriosclerosis, heart disease, gout, liver disease, gall stones, knee pain, and many other illnesses.

The Effect of Kampo on Obesity

Treatment is the same in both modern medicine and Kampo therapy. Diet therapy (limiting caloric intake) and exercise as well as drug therapy is prescribed. However, the most important thing for successful treatment is the effort of the patient. No matter how much medicine is administered, it must be understood that if the patient is not committed to the diet and exercise program, there will be no improvement.

One advantage of Kampo is that it can be used to regulate the metabolism of fats (hyperlipidism, arteriosclerosis), and thus prevent the occurrence of heart diseases. Kampo is also effective for treating other illnesses associated with obesity such as hypertension, diabetes, joint inflammation, etc.

Also, when compared to western medicine, Kampo has very few untoward effects on the digestive system and no serious side effects. It can be safely taken over long periods of time by both adults and children.

Treatment with Kampo

When using Kampo for obese patients, there are two major groups to consider. In one group, the patient is very strong, has a strong build, usually a large abdomen and thick, hard, swollen subcutaneous fat, and a tendency to get constipation. For this group, Kampo medications which remove excess stored fat are prescribed.

The other type of patient includes those who perspire easily, tire easily, are not so strong and usually have a pale complexion. These people are overweight with fluid. Although the abdomen is distended, when pressed, it is very soft and lacks muscle tone. For this group, a Kampo medication which regulates fluid metabolism is prescribed.

Actual Examples of Treatment

For those with a strong constitution, and who often tend to have hypertension and/or constipation:

BOFU-TSUSHO-SAN: For the "beer barrel" type of obesity.

DAI-SAIKO-TO: Used in cases when the epigastrium, especially the right side, is distended and painful. When pressed, the patient feels pain. The patient may have stiff shoulders, and a strong build. Also used for obesity accompanied by diabetes or hepatitis.

TOKAKU-JOKI-TO: Often used for obesity in women, when the patient feels pain upon pressure on the right under the navel, and experiences headrushes, coldness, and menstrual irregularities.

For those with a weak constitution:

BOI-OGI-TO: For patients who perspire easily, lack muscle tone, are corpulent with fluid, experience pain in the knees, and whose lower back feels heavy.

CHAPTER 10

DIABETES MELLITUS

Diabetes is caused by a lack of insulin. Insulin is a hormone secreted in the pancreas, which controls the amount of sugar in the blood. According to the amount of insulin secreted, diabetes can be divided into two types.

The first type occurs when there is absolutely no insulin secretion. This is known as "insulinopenic diabetes" (insulin dependent). With the second type, there is a large amount of sugar in the blood, despite normal or even supernormal insulin secretion, because the body is not able to make use of the insulin. This is called "insulinoplethoric diabetes" (not insulin dependent).

The Effect of Kampo on Diabetes

Modern medicine treats this disease by diet and exercise therapy in order to control the patient's obesity. For insulinopenic types, insulin injections are necessary, but insulinoplethoric types are administered diabetic drugs orally.

Unfortunately, it is necessary to control diabetes with drugs for the entire life of the patient. It is not unusual for the patient to suffer hypoglycemia as a serious side effect of taking diabeteic drugs. However, with Kampo medicines, hypoglycemia does not occur as it does when using oral diabetic drugs.

It should be noted, however, that Kampo is most appropriate for treating mild cases of insulinoplethoric diabetes. Insulinopenic cases, of course, must be administered insulin. There have been many insulinoplethoric cases where treatment with Kampo medication alone has normalized blood sugar levels and relieved listlessness, thirst, and other subjective symptoms.

Treatment with Kampo

When using Kampo, formulas are used which treat the typical symptoms of diabetes, such as drinking too much, thirst and polyuria. Some typical formulas are Byakko-Ka-Ninjin-To and Hachimi-Jio-Gan. These do lower blood sugar levels, but their action is weaker than western oral diabetic drugs.

Although the hypoglycemic mechanism of these Kampo medications is still not completely clear, the following is a brief summary of what is known at the present time:

In Byakko-Ka-Ninjin-To, there are two crude drugs which have been reported to have hypoglycemic actions in animal experiments. One of them, ginseng, is known to increase insulin secretion. Hachimi-Jio-Gan has been found to have an action which suppresses the insulin resistant hormone glycogen, and which also raises blood sugar levels. In this way, Kampo is effective in suppressing insulin hormones, in increasing insulin secretion, in strengthening the original effect of resisting the insulin itself and in stabilizing the hormone imbalance which predisposes a person to diabetes.

Actual Examples of Treatment

For cases where there is extreme thirst:

BYAKKO-KA-NINJIN-TO: For a patient with a strong constitution, sometimes with itchy skin.

For cases where there are nerve disturbances, pain in the legs and numbness:

HACHIMI-JIO-GAN: For patients with a weak constitution, thirst, loss of power from the waist down, impotence, and frequent urination at night.

GOSHA-JINKI-GAN: Same symptoms as above except that the lower back pain and nocturia are more frequent.

CHAPTER 11

COMMON COLD

The "common cold" is truly the most common of all illnesses. Yet modern medicine has still not been able to come up with any medicine which treats the actual cold itself. However, to prevent secondary infections, antibiotics are used, in addition to a variety of antifebrile-analgesics, antitussives, expectorants, and antihistamines that are usually taken to excess. Not only do these drugs fail to cure the cold itself, but they also cause problems with the digestive system, skin rashes and other annoying side effects. They should never be taken for a long period of time!

The Effect of Kampo on the Common Cold

Kampo practitioners, for nearly 2000 years, have been curing the actual cold itself in its early stages. In Kampo, much emphasis is put on the early cold symptoms such as headaches, chills and fever. When these symptoms are pronounced, a holistic judgement of the patient's weakness or strength of resistance is made. Then the most appropriate prescription is selected. If this does, indeed, match the patient's condition, symptoms disappear within 20 to 30 minutes.

In a typical case, the doctor is seen when the cold has settled in. The patient's pulse is taken. If it is weak and the inside of the patient's mouth is sticky and bitter, formulas containing bupleurum are used. If this does prove to be the correct medication, patients recover within a day or two.

Actual Examples of Treatment

KAKKON-TO: Used when patient is strong, with headache, chills, fever, stiff neck and back, has slight fever but does not perspire.

MA-KYO-KAN-SEKI-TO: Strong patient, has a fever, cough, thirst, perspires. Has cough with thin, foamy sputum, with severe sneezing, and nasal discharge.

MAO-TO: Patient is strong, has headaches, chills and fever. There is a tendency to perspire and the pulse is weak.

SHO-SAIKO-TO: Patient is weak and has had the cold for some time. The upper abdomen is distended, there is discomfort in the mouth, loss of appetite, occasional low-grade fever, and nausea.

CHIKUJO-UNTAN-TO: Weak patient. A continuous fever, frequent coughs with much phlegm, and insomnia.

CHAPTER 12

GASTRIC AND DUODENAL ULCERS

Gastric and duodenal ulcers are closely related to stomach secretions of acid and pepsin which are present when food is being digested. They are also called "peptic ulcers".

Stomach ulcers do not necessarily occur when there is an increase of "attacking" stomach acid and pepsin. There must also be an imbalance in the body's "defensive factor" for an ulcer to occur.

The ulcer defenses in the body work through two substances—an acid regulator and a stomach wall perforation blocker. Blood circulation is also often considered to be an added factor in a healthy stomach. Ulcers in young people are often caused by the attacking acid and ulcers in older people by a weakening of the defensive factor.

The upset in balance of the attacking acid and defensive factors is often due to life-style factors of stress, mental and physical fatigue, character/personality, and the overconsumption of food and alcohol. Stress plays a particularly large role in the development of ulcers. These factors influence the secretion of stomach juices, stomach movement, and blood circulation. Fever or illnesses of the central nervous system can predispose a person to ulcers.

Many patients experience the following symptoms before being hospitalized: Acute abdominal pain, pain in the epigastrium, nausea and vomiting, inflammation or hemorrhaging of the mucous membrane due to ulcers. In serious cases, the patient may vomit blood or have blood in the stools and suffer from shock. But there are also, strangely, cases where there are no severe symptoms at all. Pain may be experienced soon after eating, 2–3 hours after eating, or only on an empty stomach but lessens immediately after eating.

The Effect of Kampo on Gastric and Duodenal Ulcers

Treatment with Kampo is usually carried out in the relatively chronic stages of these illnesses. When there is hemorrhaging, perforation or adhesions, surgery is more appropriate.

Dr. Shuichi Mizuno of National Okura Hospital used only Shigyaku-San (Kampo) on elderly patients with gastric ulcers. The results, checked with an endoscope, showed that after 8 weeks, about 80% of the patients' scars were virtually healed. These figures are about the same as when histamin H2 receptor depressant, an attacking factor depressant, is used.

Treatment with Kampo

Kampo's advantage is that it can be used for elderly patients who cannot tolerate very strong drugs, and for patients who have many illnesses simultaneously and must take many different medicines. Also, the percentage of gastric ulcers that recur is high. When Kampo is used in such cases, the cure is permanent and without relapse.

With Kampo treatment, it is not necessary to find the position of the ulcer, nor to distinguish between the comparative merits and demerits of the attacking factor. Only the strength of the patient, his complexion and degree of pain are taken into account when selecting a prescription.

Actual Examples of Treatment

For cases where the effect of stress is strong and there is tendency to become depressed:

SHIGYAKU-SAN: For those with a strong feeling of anxiety, insomnia and other psychological symptoms.

SAIKO-KEISHI-TO: For those with average constitution who have nervous problems and discomfort in the epigastrium.

HANGE-SHASHIN-TO: For those with average constitution, suffering from nausea, vomiting, borborygmus, and who get diarrhea easily.

ANCHU-SAN: For patients with thin build, who are slightly weak, with heartburn, and stomach pain.

For cases where there is a tendency to be anemic from blood in the stools or from vomiting blood:

SHO-KENCHU-TO: Patient is weak, tires easily, has pale complexion, and abdominal pain.

SHIKUNSHI-TO: Same as the above, except that all these symptoms are more severe.

CHAPTER 13

IRRITABLE BOWEL SYNDROME

IBS is often found in developed countries such as the United States. It is caused by stress. When stress disturbs the autonomic nervous system, the rhythm of the colon and secretion function is upset, causing abdominal pain, discomfort in the lower abdomen, a feeling of distension in the abdomen, borborygmus, diarrhea, constipation and other intestinal symptoms. Other symptoms also occur, such as fatigue, headaches, palpitations, night sweat and insomnia. Diarrhea that is caused by organic disorders or bacterial infection is not treated as IBS. Abdominal pain, diarrhea and constipation due to IBS are so frequent that IBS is a great hindrance to daily life in big cities.

According to the definition developed by American doctors, the various types of IBS are: "spastic colon," "mucous colon," "colonic neurosis," and "nervous indigestion." The causes range from stress and other psychological factors to physical factors such as the abuse of laxatives, irregular bowel emptying, and excessive cigarette smoking.

IBS tends to occur in patients between the ages of 30 and 50, and more so in men than in women. According to Cecil's text on internal medicine, IBS accounts for 50% of all digestive system complaints. (This figure is about 30% in Japan.)

Upon palpation of the abdomen near the colon (especially the S-shaped colon in the lower left abdomen), a lump or pain is often felt. There may also be a rumbling in the abdomen due to gas in the intestine.

The Effect of Kampo on IBS

In Kampo, treatment is carried out according to constipation and diarrhea type. In cases where both occur, treatment is prescribed based on the most usual complaint. In modern western medicine, there are many ways of treatment but most doctors use tranquilizers. When there is abdominal pain, anticolon drugs are used. When there is diarrhea and constipation, intestine-regulating drugs are used.

In Japan many university related hospitals, under the guidance of professors specializing in the digestive system, have reported that treatment of neurotic digestive disorders including IBS has been more effective when Kampo rather than western medicine was used.

Also, it was reported that the patients treated with Kampo medications tended to have very few side effects and less possibility of relapse after stopping treatment.

Treatment with Kampo

When cases of IBS are analyzed from the point of view of Asian medicine, the people with the following peculiarities predominate.

1) XU sho (kyo sho): those with a weakened constitution.
2) Cold sho: Coldness of the waist and legs, with symptoms worsening in the winter and under cold circumstances.
3) Those with psychological and nervous symptoms, insomnia, anxiety, fatigue, etc.

Many times, these symptoms all occur together in a patient. This is referred to as IBS clinical pneumonia.

In Kampo, the body's overall condition is strengthened. In addition, the emotional condition of the patient is stabilized with prescriptions containing the proper combinations of crude drugs.

Actual Examples of Treatment

When constipation is the main symptom:

KEISHI-KA-SHAKUYAKU-TO: Patient relatively weak. Abdomen is always distended with abdominal pain.

KEISHI-KA-SHAKUYAKU-DAIO-TO: Same symptoms as the above, but constipation is more severe.

When diarrhea is the main symptom:

HANGE-SHASHIN-TO: Average constitution. Experiences nausea or vomiting, borborygmus.

NINJIN-TO: Weak. Body feels tired. Vertigo and cold extremities.

CHAPTER 14

MALAISE OF THE URINARY TRACT

In these cases, although there are usually no abnormalities found functionally or in urinary tests, the patient has symptoms of general malaise, such as polyuria and discomfort in the lower abdomen. In general, these symptoms occur after acute or chronic cystitis. Although the bacterial infection has been treated successfully, the symptoms mentioned above often persist.

The Effect of Kampo on General Malaise of the Urinary Tract

In general, although Kampo's antibacterial properties are not as quick acting as modern antibiotics, they often prove highly effective in treating this problem. When Kampo is used along with western medicine, the results are even better than when treated with modern drugs alone.

Actual Examples of Treatment

CHOREI-TO: Used for polyuria, feeling of incomplete urination, pain upon urination, hematuria.

GORIN-SAN: For average constitution with urethritis which has become chronic. Difficulty in urinating, pain upon urinating, hematuria.

RYUTAN-SHAKAN-TO: For strong constitution. Inflammation of the urinary organs with pain upon urinating, polyuria, leukorrhea.

SEISHIN-RENSHI-IN: For patients with weak digestive system and weak constitution. Difficulty in urinating, incomplete urination, pain upon urination.

CHOREI-TO-GO-SHIMOTSU-TO: Same as above, except that the symptoms have become complicated. Polyuria, pain upon urinating, incomplete urinating, chronic hematuria.

CHAPTER 15

MYOMA OF THE UTERUS

This is most common of all benign tumors. There may be only one tumor or there may be many. In general, the tumors are hard and range from the size of the tip of the small finger to much larger. Their exact cause has not yet been determined. The tumors seldom appear before adolescence. The main symptoms are copious menstruation, dismenorrhea, irregular hemorrhaging of the urogenital organs, leukorrhea and infertility.

The Effect of Kampo on Myoma of the Uterus

Fortunately, myomas are benign, and Kampo is very effective in treating the symptoms of pain in the lower abdomen and back, and copious menstruation. It is also effective in treating less frequent symptoms such as tinnitis, loss of appetite, nausea, vertigo, insomnia, swollen breasts, constipation, and a heavy head. It is very effective in treating the symptoms, although its effect in reducing the size of the myoma is negligible. Therefore, Kampo does not supercede surgery. However, the help it gives women is indeed welcome and does not involve removing the uterus.

Actual Examples of Treatment

KEISHI-BUKURYO-GAN: Patient usually has a good build and a ruddy complexion. Abdomen is distended, with resistance in lower abdomen.

TOKAKU-JOKI-TO: Strong build and strong constitution. Has headrushes with constipation.

UNKEI-TO: Weak constitution. Hotness of the palms of the hands, dry lips, and coldness and pain in the lower abdomen.

NYOSHIN-SAN: Average constitution. Nervous problems including anxiety, insomnia, headaches and vertigo that accompany menstruation or menopause.

CHAPTER 16

NASAL ALLERGIES

Nasal allergies usually harass us in the early spring or autumn, or when we are working about the house. Nose and eyes become itchy, there is sneezing, watery nasal discharge, and the nose may become blocked. Other symptoms, such as the loss of the sense of smell, headaches and tearing may also appear.

This illness is frequent in people who have inherited allergy-causing factors, and who have antibodies to a substance in pollen, house dust, etc. (antigen). As a result of the reaction between the antigen and antibodies, beginning with histamines, chemical transmitters are released which cause the symptoms to appear.

The Effect of Kampo on Nasal Allergies

The main symptom of nasal allergies are frequent sneezing and copious watery nasal discharge. These irregularities in fluid discharge correspond to what is known in Kampo as "Suidoku". Sho-seiryu-To is the Kampo medicine often used when these symptoms are present. Not only does this stop the runny nose and sneezing, but it may also lead to a complete cure of the allergy. Allergy sufferers should use Kampo and also avoid breathing in pollen, dust and other antigen-containing substances.

Actual Examples of Treatment

KAKKON-TO: For cases with stiff neck and headaches, frequent attacks of sneezing and nasal discharge.

BAKUMONDO-TO: Severe sneezing, but little nasal discharge. Cough with difficulty in coughing up phlegm.

SAIKO-KEISHI-KANKYO-TO: Pale complexion, tends to sweat easily above the neck.

CHAPTER 17

LUMBAGO (Lower Back Pain)

Lumbago is not in itself a name of an illness, but is the name given to the symptom of pain in the lower back. The causes of this pain cover a wide area. Muscular fatigue, irregularities of the back bone and disease are a few. Also, neuralgia, tumors, cancer, or sprains and broken bones may also be contributing factors.

The three types of lumbago are: muscular, muscular membrane types and static lumbago. The character of their pathology cannot be found.

The Effect of Kampo on Lumbago

Once again, compared to the effect of western drugs, the action of Kampo is comparatively weak. When the pain is severe, other strong drugs should be prescribed immediately.

However, Kampo does relieve the pain by regulating the functional disturbances that afflict the patient. Treatment with Kampo is also highly useful in eliminating the symptoms which may accompany lumbago: coldness, headrushes, stiff shoulders, vertigo, and fatigue. In addition, in cases where lumbago has become chronic and drugs are used habitually, Kampo drugs can be substituted safely because of their freedom from side effects.

Treatment with Kampo

Kampo treatment is usually reserved for lumbago caused by functional disorders. Although there may be mechanical pressure confirmed by tests causing the lumbago, this is often not the only cause of pain. In such cases, surgery can be avoided and conservative Kampo treatment substituted. Chronic lumbago is especially suited for Kampo. Diet and lifestyle are also important factors in such cases.

Actual Examples of Treatment

For elderly people with fatigue, thirst and weakness of the lower abdomen:
HACHIMI-JIO-GAN: For patients with weak constitution, but no digestive problems.
GOSHA-JINKI-GAN: For the same patients, but with more severe symptoms.

For cases where there are gynecological problems with pain upon pressure in the abdomen, headaches, stiff shoulders, headrushes, vertigo, coldness:
KEISHI-BUKURYO-GAN: For patients with strong constitution.
TOKAKU-JOKI-TO: For patients with strong constitution suffering from constipation, anxiety, insomnia and other nervous conditions.

In patients who, from the waist down to the legs, have muscle pain, joint pain, neuralgia, tendency to edema and experiencing pain upon pressure in the lower abdomen.
SOKEI-KAKKETSU-TO: For those with an average constitution.

For cases with coldness of the extremities due to poor circulation in the peripheral blood vessels:
TOKI-SHIGYAKU-KA-GOSYUYU-SHOKYO-TO: For those with very weak constitution.

For cases with pain and swelling of the joints of the extremities and an impediment in movement:
KEISHI-KA-JUTSUBU-TO: For those with weak constitution.

Where there is severe coldness of the lower back and legs and copious urine:
RYO-KYO-JUTSU-KAN-TO: For those with weak constitution.

CHAPTER 18

PSORIASIS

Psoriasis is a skin disease which has peculiar silvery, white scales. Although it does not usually affect the general condition of the body, it is very difficult to treat and usually becomes chronic. Psoriasis mainly affects Caucasians, but it is also on the increase in Japan.

The Effect of Kampo on Psoriasis

The orthodox treatment for psoriasis includes PUVA therapy, Mettotorekisa-To, and steroid hormones. If these treatments are used for any length of time, there is the danger of serious side effects. Therefore, this is a most difficult disease for doctors to treat. Accordingly, more and more patients are turning to Kampo. Western doctors are turning to Kampo, also, to discover its secrets. They find:

- As opposed to the localized therapy used by western medicine, Kampo helps to regulate the balance of the body, build up the constitution, and also acts as a preventative.
- Compared to western medicine, there are very few side effects. Kampo may therefore be used for long periods of time.
- When Kampo is used along with strong modern drugs, it helps to reduce the side effects of the drugs and also gives a generally better result than expected from western drugs alone.

Actual Examples of Treatment

KEISHI-BUKURYO-GAN and UNSEI-IN: The first is an anti-blood stagnation formula and has effects that western drugs do not have. It is used effectively in all cases where there is blood stagnation.

OREN-GEDOKU-TO and UNSEI-IN: Tests show that these two Kampo treatments may prevent psoriasis and that through their use dangerous steroid treatments may not be needed. The high effectiveness of Kampo for various skin diseases (chronic urturcaria, etc.) gives much hope for the future.

CHAPTER 19

HEMORRHOIDS

What are Hemorrhoids?

These "piles" generally occur around the anus. They are classified as follows: 1) Those caused by bad blood circulation; 2) Those caused by bacteria; and 3) Those caused by external injuries or mechanical malfunctions such as lacerated anus.

The Effect of Kampo on Hemorrhoids

Kampo is recommended highly for piles and anal fissures. Piles result from stagnant blood in the veins of the rectum. Constipation, fatigue, stress, alcohol and smoking also aggravate this condition.

Kampo practitioners use anti-blood stagnation medicines to treat hemorrhoids. Not only do they treat the condition, but they also carefully assess the patient's whole physical condition and balance. If a person's state of health is in poor equilibrium, morbidity may also be restored to normal. Kampo is most effective in the treatment of those hemorrhoids caused by poor blood circulation and by bacteria. Complete cures are effected when the patient maintains a regular life style, reduces alcohol and cigarette use, and takes hot baths.

Actual Examples of Treatment

OTSUJI-TO: Average constitution, with constipation.

KEISHI-BUKURYO-GAN: For strong constitution, with pain upon pressure in lower abdomen.

DAIO-BOTAMPI-TO: For strong constitution.

KYUKI-KYOGAI-TO: For continuous hemorrhaging.

Also anti-blood stagnation prescriptions plus Otsuji-To (Hochu-Ekki-To).

External:
OTSUJI-TO plus anti-blood stagnation prescriptions.
(Anti-blood stagnation formulas: Tokaku-Joki-To, Keishi-Bukuryo-Gan, Daio-Botanpi-To)

Anal fissures:
OTSUJI-TO plus anti-blood stagnation prescriptions.

PART FOUR

Kampo Manual

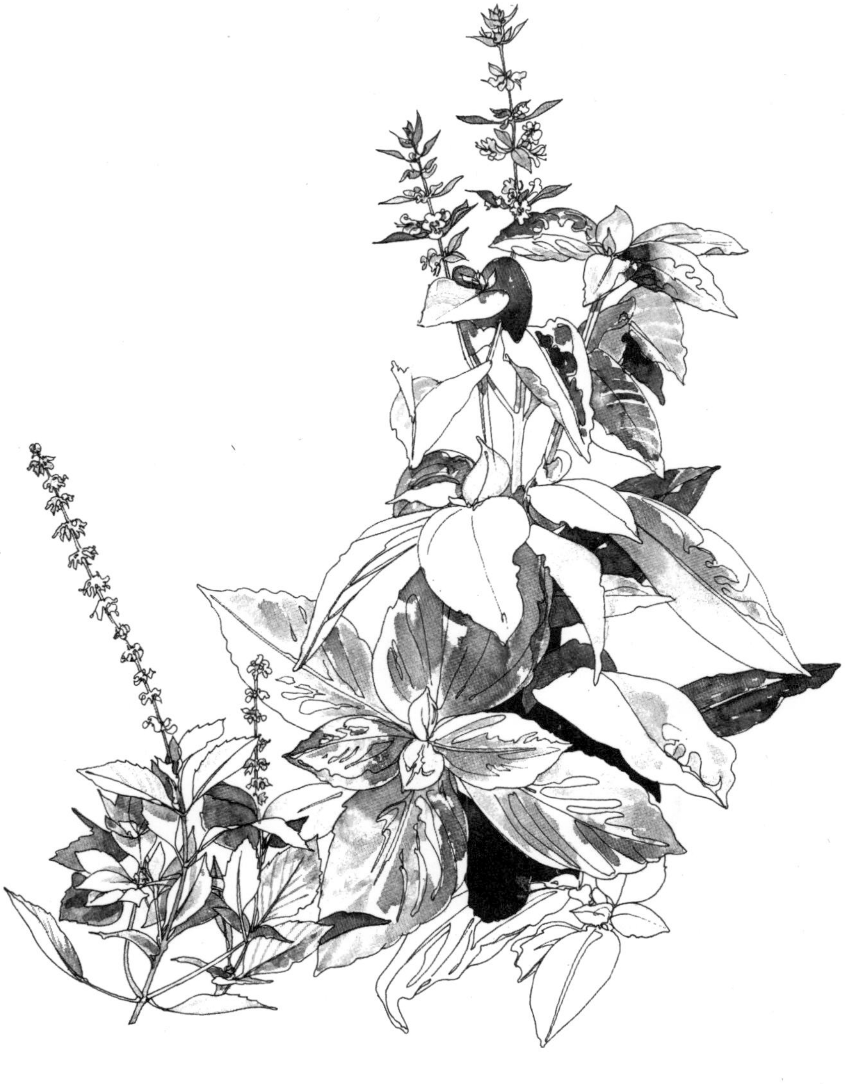

"The Great Spirit is our father, but the earth is our mother.
She nourishes us, and healing plants she gives us."

—Big Thunder, North American Indian

INTRODUCTION TO UNREFINED DRUGS

The crude drugs listed in this section are those folk medicines still commonly used in Kampo.

The botanical name, directly under the common name in Latin, is a world-wide standard for precise identification. A few lines of general background information about each plant are given next. To investigate each herb thoroughly is, of course, the work of a lifetime. In my own case it has become a passion. Working with herbs gives one the opportunity to unravel some of the great mysteries of nature and to understand the most elemental forces of the universe. How can such a search be anything but rewarding?

The pharmacological properties listed next refer to those properties found through research in Japan and recorded in medical journals. Due to space limitations, it is not necessarily complete. However, it will give the reader a general idea of how each drug works in the human system.

The reference to Japanese medical classics will also give the reader some idea of how each drug has been used in traditional Kampo. Note: Because some of the terms in the originals do not exist in English, the translator has given them their nearest possible meaning in contemporary language. Following are the Japanese medical classics from which our information has been drawn:

Yakucho (Characteristics of Medicine) by Todo Yoshimasu. 1771.
Yakucho Zokuhen (Characteristics of Medicine, Supplemental Volume) by Kotozan Murai. 1778.
Ippondo-Yakusen (Selected Medicines) by Shuan Kagawa (Pen Name *Ippondo*). 1734.
Ippondo-Yakusen-Zokuhen (Supplementary Volume to the *Ippondo-Yakusen*) by Shuan Kagawa. 1738.
Koho-Yakugi (Discussion on Medicines from the Works of Zhang Zong-Jing) by Sohaku Asada. 1836.
Koho-Yakugi-Zokuhen (Supplementary Volume to the *Koho-Yakugi*) by Sakumin Uzuse. 1870.

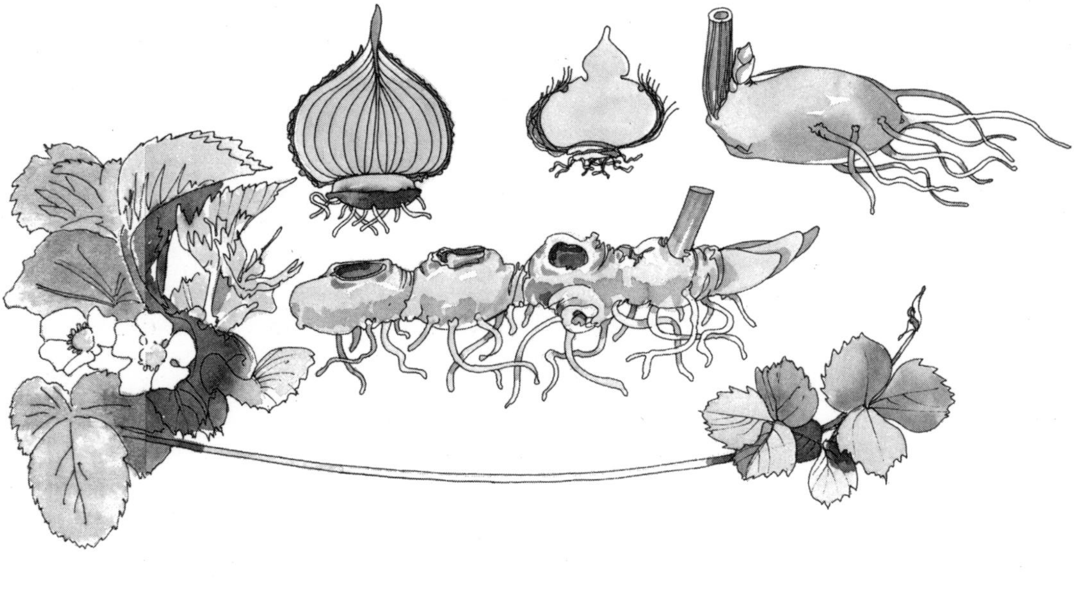

NOTE: *Herbs are so well-known and easily available that there is a strong, natural tendency to use them without professional advice. This can be dangerous if illness persists for a long time, or becomes severe. In such cases, a doctor should be consulted at once.*

UNREFINED DRUGS

附 子

ACONITE

Ranuculaceae. *Aconitum carmichaeli Debx.*
Common name: Aconite, Monk's hood, wolfbane
Japanese pronunciation: Bushi

Background: Aconite is considered the most Yang of all Oriental herbs and can be toxic if used to excess. According to myth, saliva from the mouth of the three-headed dog that guards Hades once fell on aconite, making it a deadly poison. Hunters once tipped their arrows in aconite to kill wolves. (Hence the name wolfbane).

KAMPO: The processed root of aconite is used. (*Aconiti tuber*)

Main constituents are: Alkaloids: aconitine, mesconitine, aconine, hypaconitins, jessaconitine, atisine, songorine, kobusine, ignavine, napelline, hiegenamine (de-demethylcoclaurine), coryneine, yokonoside, etc.

Pharmacological properties: Analgesic, cardiotonic, anti-inflammatory, anti-stress ulcer, dilates the blood vessels, increases liver protein metabolism.

Usage according to Japanese classics: Used mainly to treat irregularities of the fluid metabolism. Also used to treat chills, general pain, pain in the extremities and joints, cold extremities, abdominal pain, heavy feeling in the body, spermatorrhea, nocturnal emission, and diarrhea. (Yakucho)

Used in Kampo prescriptions:
Keishi-Ka-Jutsubu-To, Gosha-Jinki-Gan, Shimbu-To, Dai-Bofu-To, Hachimi-Jio-Gan, Mao-Bushi-Saishin-To.

木 通

AKEBIA

Lardizabalaceae. *Akebia quinata* Decame.
Common name: Five-leaf Akebia
Japanese pronunciation: Mokutsū

Background: This plant has been found to be highly effective in promoting lactation when brewed together with pork knuckles.

KAMPO: The caulis of this plant is used. (*Akebiae Caulis*)

Main constituents are: Saponins: akeboside Stb, Stc, Std, Ste, akebin, aristolosids, etc. Other: potassium salt.

Pharmacological properties: Diuretic, anti-inflammatory, anti-peptic ulcer, reduces cholesterol.

Usage according to Japanese classics: Diuretic. Lubricates the joints and nine orifices (eyes, ears, nose, mouth, anus, and urethra). Relieves gonorrhea, urinary tract, edema due to disorders of the circulatory system, jaundice, and lack of breast milk. (*Ippondo-Yakusen*)

Used in Kampo prescriptions:
Gorin-San, Shofu-San, Tsu-Do-San, Toki-Shakuyaku-Ka-Goshyuyu-Shokyo-To, Ryutan-Shakan-To.

牛 膝

AMERANTHUS

Amaranthaceas. *Achryanthes fauriei Lev. et Van* 'T or *A. bidentata. Bl.*
Common name: Amaranthus
Japanese pronunciation: Goshitsu

Background: This herb has a wide distribution from China to India and Indonesia. In the past it has been used to promote circulation, dissolve clots, as a diuretic, and as a tonic to liver and kidneys, sinews and bones.

KAMPO: The root is used. (*Achyranthis Radix*) Main constituents are: Saponin, inokosterone, β-sitosterol, stigmasterol, amino acids, sugars.

Pharmacological properties: Anti-allergic.

Usage according to Japanese classics: Used to relieve painful and stiff joints, inflammation of urethra, hot and painful feeling upon urination, hematuria, pain of the sexual organs, irregular menstruation and other blood stagnation problems. Not to be used after stillbirth and during pregnancy. (*Ippondo-Yakusen*)

Used in Kampo prescriptions:
Gosha-Jinki-Gan, Sokei-Kakketsu-To,
Dai-Bofu-To.

知 母

ANEMARRHENA

Liliaceae. *Anemarrhena asphodeloides* Bge.
Common name: Anemarrhena
Japanese pronunciation: Chimo

Background: This herb was traditionally used in China for ailments of the lungs, stomach, and kidneys. They found it incompatible with iron preparations.

KAMPO: The rhizome of this plant is used. (*Anemarrhenae Rhizoma*)

Main constituents are: Saponins: sarsasapogenin 3-o-β-timobioside (timosaponin A-111), sarsasapogenin 3-o-β-timobioside (timosaponin A-1), etc.
Glycosides: chimonin (=magiferin), isomangiferin, etc. Vitamins: nicotinic acid, pantothenic acid.

Pharmacological properties: Anti-pyretic, hypoglycemic, anti-peptic ulcer, inhibits cyclic AMP.

Usage according to Japanese classics: Used mainly to treat hotness of the extremities and fever with discomfort. (*Yakucho-Zokuhen*)

Used in Kampo prescriptions:
Sansonin-To, Jiin-Koka-To, Jiin-Shiho-To, Shofu-San, Shin'i-Seihai-To, Byakko-Ka-Ninjin-To.

白芷

ANGELICA

Umbelliferae *Angelica dahurica* Benth. et Hook.
Common name: Angelica, Master wort
Japanese pronunciation: Byakushi

Background: Angelica is a standout in more ways than one. It towers over all other plants in an herb garden. Legend has it that in the 17th century, in a year of great plague, an angel told the fearful populace to take angelica to protect themselves from infection. The herb's aromatic, bitter-sweet taste commends itself into the stomach, easing indigestion, colic, and flatulence. Angelica is also antibacterial and antifungal. Pinene, a component of the oil, is also an expectorant. The plant's antispasmodic action makes it effective in treating menstrual periods.

Caution: Wild angelica has several poisonous lookalikes.

KAMPO: The root of this plant is used. (*Angelicae Dahuricae Radix*)

Main constituents are: Croumarin derivatives: byak-angelicol, imperatorin, oxypuecedanin.

Pharmacological properties: Central nervous system stimulant, interferon inducer.

Usage according to Japanese classics: Used mainly to treat stagnant pathogens accompanied by headaches, and hard, painful swellings of the face. (*Yakucho-Zokuhen*)

Used in Kampo prescriptions:
Keigai-Rengyo-To, Goshaku-San, Sei-Jo-Bofu-To, Senkyu-Chacho-San, Sokei-Kakketsu-To.

当 帰

ANGELICA (Tang-kuei)

Umbelliferae *Angelica acutiloba* KITAGAWA
Common name: Angelica, Tang-kuei
Japanese pronunciation: Tōki

Main constituents: Essential oils: ligustilide, n-butylidenphthalide, sedanonic acid, safrol. Fatty acids: palmitic acid, linolic acid. Croumarin derivatives: bergaptene, scopoletin. Polyethylene components: falcarinol, falcarindiol. Others: vitamin B_{12}, nicotinic acid.

Pharmacological properties: Central nervous system suppressant, antitussive, antipyretic, muscle relaxant, hypotensive, dilates the peripheral blood vessels, anti-coagulant, anti-inflammatory, anti-allergy, immunomoderating, anti-tumor.

Usage according to Japanese classics: Used to resolve blood activities, drainage of pus: improves blood stagnation and maintains essential body fluids. Also used to treat pain from red and swollen eyes, resolves body after childbirth, rids old blood, and resolves irregular bleeding from genital organs, also improves infected swellings (boils, tumors, etc.) from within. (*Yakucho*)

Used in Kampo prescriptions:
Unkei-To, Unsei-To, Otsuji-To, Kami-Kihi-To, Kami-Shoyo-San, Kihi-To, Kyuki-Kyogai-To, Keigai-Rengyo-To, Goshaku-San, Gorin-San, Saiko-Seikan-To, Jiin-Koka-To, Jiin-Shiho-To, Shiun-Ko, Shichimotsu-Koka-To, Shimotsu-To, Juzen-Taiho-To, Juncho-To, Shofu-San, Seisho-Ekki-To, Seihai-To, Sokei-Kakketsu-To, Tsu-Do-San, Toki-Inshi, Toki-Kenchu-To, Toki-Shigyaku-Ka-Gosyuyu-Shokyo-To, Toki-Shakuyaku-San, Toki-To, Nyoshin-San, Ninjin-Yoei-To, Bofu-Tsusho-San, Hochu-Ekki-To, Yokuinin-To, Yoku-Kan-San, Yoku-Kan-San-Ka-Chimpi-Hange, Ryutan-Shakan-To.

杏 仁

APRICOT

Rosaceae, *Prunus armeniaca* L., var. ANUS MAXIM.
Common name: Apricot
Japanese pronunciation: Kyōnin

Background: Apricots are rich in iron and minerals and therefore are traditionally used in folk medicine to treat anemia. They are also frequently used as a laxative.

KAMPO: The kernels of the fruit are used. (*armeniacae Semen*)

Main constituents are: Hydrocyanic glycocides: amygdalin, etc. Fatty oils: oleic acid. Steroids: estrone, estradiol 17-β, etc. Others: emulsion.

Pharmacological properties: Follicle hormone-like action.

Usage according to Japanese classics: Used mainly to treat fluid and mucous which have become stagnant in chest. Also used to treat stridor, coughing, shortness of breath, pain and distension of the epigastrium, chest pain, and edema. (*Yakucho*)

Used in Kampo prescriptions:
Goko-To, Juncho-To, Shimpi-To, Seihai-To, Mao-To, Ma-Kyo-Kan-Seki-To, Ma-Kyo-Yoku-Kan-To, Mashinin-Gan, Ryo-Kan-Kyo-Mi-Shin-Ge-Nin-To.

白 朮

ATRACTYLODES (Japonica)

Compositae, *Atractylodes japonica* KOIDZUMI
Common name: Atractylodes
Japanese pronunciation: Byakujutsu

Background: This plant has been used in China, Korea, and Japan because of its affinity for the spleen and stomach. Aids in cases of diarrhea, nausea and vomiting, leukorrhea, gastroenteritis, aching joints and muscles, weakness and sluggishness.

KAMPO: The skinned root of this plant is used. (*Atractylodes Rhizoma*)

Main constituents are: Essential oils: atractylon atractylenoline I, II, III.

Pharmacological properties: Diuretic, hypoglycemic, anticoagulant, hepatoprotective, anti-peptic ulcer, anti-inflammatory, interferon inducing.

Usage according to Japanese classics: Used mainly to treat fluid imbalance and irregularities of the fluid metabolism. Also used to treat polyuria, dysuria, discomfort and pain, phlegm, coughing, vomiting, spermatorrhea, hood vertigo, diarrhea, the vomiting and dribbling of saliva. (*Yakucho*)

Used in Kampo prescriptions:
Irei-To-Kihi-To, Jiin-Shiho-To, Nijutsu-To, Ninjin-Yoei-To, Hange-Byakujutsu-Temma-To, Bofu-Tsusho-San, Ryo-Kyo-Jutsu-Kan-To.

蒼 朮

ATRACTYLODES

Compositae, *Atractylodes Lancea* DC
Common name: Atractyloidea, thistle type
Japanese pronunciation: Sōjutsu

Background: (See *Atractylodes japonica*.) This is a related plant with different uses.

KAMPO: The rhizome of this plant is used. (*Atractylodis Lanceae Rhizoma*)

Main constituents are: Essential oils: hinesol, β-eudesmol, elemol, atractylodin.

Pharmacological properties: Anti-peptic ulcer, cholagogous, hypoglycemic, antibacterial. Accelerates the electrolyte metabolism.

Usage according to Japanese classics: Used mainly to treat irregularities of the fluid metabolism. Relieves dysuria, polyuria, pain and discomfort, fluid irregularities (stridor with phlegm, vomiting, etc), spermatorrhea, nocturnal discharge of semen, hood vertigo, diarrhea, vomiting and dribbling of saliva. (*Yakucho*)

Used in Kampo prescriptions:
Irei-To-Kihi-To, Inchin-Gorei-San, Eppi-Ka-Justu-To, Kami-Kihi-To, Kami-Shoyo-San, Keishi-Ka-Jutsubu-To, Keishi-Ninjin-To, Goshaku-San, Gorei-San, Sairei-To, Jiin-Koka-To, Shikunshi-To, Juzen-Taiho-To, Shofu-San, Shimbu-To, Seisho-Ekki-To, Sokei-Kakketsu-To, Dai-Bofu-To, Ji-Zuso-Ippo, Toki-Shakuyaku-San, Nijutsu-To, Nyoshin-San, Ninjin-To, Bukuryo-In, Bukuryo-In-Go-Hange-Koboku-To, Heii-San, Boi-Ogi-To, Hochu-Ekki-To, Yokuinin-To, Yoku-Kan-San, Yoku-Kan-San-Ka-Chimpi-Hange, Rikkunshi-To, Ryo-Kei-Jutsu-Kan-To.

竹 茹

BAMBOO

Gramineae, *Phyllostachys nigra* Munro var. *henosis* Stapf ex Rendle or P. *bambusoides* Sieb. et Zucc.
Common name: Bamboo
Japanese pronunciation: Chikujo

Background: What would man do without bamboo? In the Far East it is used for 1,001 uses: building and making rafts, paper, deodorant, and as a vegetable. Therefore, it is not at all surprising that it was found to have medicinal properties as well.

KAMPO: In Japan, shavings of the inner stem of this plant are used. (*Phyllostachysis Caulis in Taeniam*)

Main constituents are: Triterpenoids: arundoin, cylindrin, taraxerol, friedelin. Others: sugars, amino acids, vitamins.

Pharmacological properties: Central nervous system suppressant. Anti-inflammatory, anti-tumor, inhibits cyclic AMP.

Usage according to Japanese classics: Used to relieve vomiting and nausea, chills, fever, and respiratory illnesses accompanied by a reduction in lung function and blood in the sputum. Also used for patients recovering from infectious disease. (*Koho-Yakugi*)

Used in Kampo prescriptions:
Chikujo-Untan-To, Seihai-To.

麦 芽

BARLEY

Gramineae, *Hordeum vulgare* L. var. *hexastion* ASCHERS
Common name: Barley
Japanese pronunciation: Bakuga

Background: In China, the herb was considered to have abortifacient properties which facilitate contractions during childbirth. It was also considered to promote digestion and the movement of grains and vegetables through the system.

KAMPO: The dried sprouts of this plant are used. (*Hordei Fructus Germinatus*)

Main Constituents: Starches, proteins, maltose, vitamins.

Used in Kampo prescriptions:
Hange-Byakujutsu-Temma-To.

蘇 葉

BEEFSTEAK PLANT

Labiatae, *Perilla frutescens* Britt. var. acuta Kudo.
Common name: Beefsteak plant
Japanese pronunciation: Soyo (Shiso)

Background: This is an ancient Chinese remedy used for thousands of years as a sedative and to fight infection.

KAMPO: The leaves of this plant are used in Kampo. (*Perillae Herba*)

Main constituents are: Pigments: Antocyan pigment. Essential oils: perillaldehyde, e-limonene, menthol.

Pharmacological properties: Sedative, immunomoderating, antibacterial.

Usage according to Japanese classics: Although its effects are weak, it expels pathogens from the body's epidermis, helps the circulation of ch'i, and relieves discomfort of the epigastrium. (*Ippondo-Yakusen*)

Used in Kampo prescriptions:
Koso-San, Saiboku-To, Jinso-In,
Shimpi-To, Hange-Koboku-To,
Bukuryo-In-Go-Hange-Koboku-To.

檳榔子

BETEL NUT

Palmae, *areca catechu* L.
Common name: Betel nut
Japanese pronunciation: Binrōji

Background: In the West, the betel nut was made famous by Michener's "Tales of the South Pacific." Natives delight in it because it is a stimulant that gives a feeling of well-being, aids digestion, sweetens the breath, and strengthens the gums. It also promotes the secretion of saliva and intestinal juices. Recently, scientists have discovered that it can destroy tape worms, and cure problems of the urinary tract. In large doses it can have a toxic effect.

KAMPO: The nut is used in Kampo. (*Arecae Semen*)

Main constituents are: Alkaloids: arecoline, arecaidine, arecolidine, guvacine, gavacoline. Steroids: diosgenin, β-sitosterol. Other: tannin, gallic acid, amino acids, pigments, and essential oils.

Pharmacological properties: Stimulates the central nervous system and parasympathetic nervous system.

Usage according to Japanese classics: Aids digestion and unblocks stagnant food from the digestive tract. (*Ippondo-Yakusen*)

Used in Kampo prescription:
Nyoshin-San.

升 麻

BLACK COHOSH

Ranunculaceae, *Cimicifuga simplex* Wormsk.
Common name: Black cohosh, bugbane.
Japanese pronunciation: Shōma

Background: The strong odor of the flowers of this plant act as an insect repellant. The hardy rootstock can be used for a variety of medical purposes including relief from headaches, tinnitis, and high blood pressure. A brew made from it is a favored Indian remedy for menstrual cramps and the pains of childbirth. As poultice it is used as a remedy for snakebite. In the 19th century, a tincture from the rhizome was helpful in treating rheumatism and neuralgia. Laboratory tests now confirm that it does have an anti-inflammatory effect. Large doses can cause symptoms of poisoning so this plant is another that must always be used with great care.

KAMPO: The rhizome is used in Kampo. (*Cimicifugae Rhizoma*)

Main constituents are: Triterpines: cimigenol, dahurinol, acerinol, cimicifugoside, cimifugenin. Steroids: β-sitosterol, stigmasterol. Other: cimifugin, norvisnagin, viusnagin, isoferulic acid, ferulic acid.

Pharmacological properties: Analgesic, sedative, antispasmodic, antipyretic, suppresses anal ulcers, anti-inflammatory, hepatoprotective, immune-suppressant, interferon inducing.

Usage according to Japanese classics: Used to treat various swellings caused by cold, heat and wind. To treat sore throat, stomatitis, bad breath, and purulent skin diseases. (*Koho-Yakugi*)

Used in Kampo prescription:
Otsuji-To, Shoma-Kakkon-To, Shin'i-Seihai-To, Hochu-Ekki-To, Rikko-San.

柴 胡

BUPLEURUM

Umbelliferae, *Bupleurum falactum*, L.
Common name: Bupleurum, Hare's Ear
Japanese pronunciation: Saiko

Background: Bupleurum is regarded as one of the finest herbs for detoxifying the liver. In Europe and Asia it is used as an antipyretic, analgesic, anti-nauseant, and relaxant. It relieves anxiety and dizziness, strengthens the eyes and limbs, and tones up the leg muscles.

KAMPO: The root is used. (*Bupleuri Radix*)

Main constituents are: Saponins: saikosaponin, a, c, d, e, f. Sterols: α-spinasterol, stigmasterol. Fatty acids: palmitic acid, stearic acid, oleic acid, linoleic acid, lignoceric acid. Other: adonitol, *l*-anomalin, arginine.

Pharmacological properties: Central nervous system suppressant, smooth muscle relaxant, anti-peptic ulcer, hepatoprotective, anti-inflammatory, anti-allergic. Inhibits cyclic AMP, prevents side effects from steroids, improves the metabolism of fats, anti-stress, interferon inducing.

Usage according to Japanese classics: Used mainly to treat tenderness and distention of the hypochondrium. Also to treat alternating chills and fever, abdominal pain and discomfort and tightness of the epigastrium. (*Yakucho*)

Used in Kampo prescription:
Otsuji-To, Kami-Kihi-To, Kami-Shoyo-San, Keigai-Rengyo-To, Saikan-To, Saiko-Keishi-To, Saiko-Keishi-Kankyo-To, Saiko-Seikan-To, Saiko-Ka-Ryukotsu-Borei-To, Sairei-To, Jiin-Shiho-To, Shigaku-San, Jumi-Haidoku-To, Sho-Saiko-To, Sho-Saiko-To-Ka-Kikyo-Sekko, Shimpi-To, Dai-Saiko-To, Chikujo-Untan-To, Hochu-Ekki-To, Yoku-Kan-San, Yoku-Kan-San-Ka-Chimpi-Hange.

麻子仁

CANNABIS

Moraceae, *Cannabis sativa* L.
Common name: Cannabis (marihuana)
Japanese pronunciation: Mashinin

Background: Marihuana was listed in the ancient pharmacopeias of China for its ability to ease pain, induce sleep, and soothe a variety of nervous disorders. In Europe, medieval physicians prescribed it to alleviate the agonies of gout. Today, marihuana is being tested as a treatment for asthma, epileptic seizures and the nausea caused by radiation therapy. This plant also has a dark side and should never be taken except under a doctor's supervision. (It is illegal or regulated in many countries.)

KAMPO: The seeds are used. (*Cannabidis Semen*)

Main constituents are: Fatty oils: olein, linolein, linelenin. Sugars: pentosan, dextrin. Other: trigonelline, choline, emulsin.

Pharmacological properties: Hypoglycemic.

Usage according to Japanese classics: Aids blood circulation; helps metabolism in various organs of the body. Relieves inflammation of the large intestine, stagnant stools, red urine due to fever, and painful urination with fever. (*Koho-Yakugi*)

Used in Kampo prescription:
Sha-Kanzo-To, Juncho-To, Mashinin-Gan.

縮砂

CARDAMON

Zingeberaceae, *Amomum xanthiodes* Wall.
Common name: Cardamom
Japanese pronunciation: Shukusha

Background: Used in Southern China originally for problems with the spleen and kidneys. Builds up bones and sinews; inhibits excess urination; antidiarrhetic; astringent; stomachic.

KAMPO: Clumps of seeds are used. (*Amomi Semen*)

Main constituents are: Essential oils: δ-camphor, δ-borneol, bornyl acetate, linalool, nerolidol. Other: liquiritin, glucovanillic acid, etc.

Pharmacological properties: Inhibits the production of prostaglandin.

Used in Kampo prescription:
Anchu-San.

菊花

CHRYSANTHEMUM

Compositae, *Chrysanthemum indicum* L.
Common name: Chrysanthemum
Japanese pronunciation: Kikka

Background: Both wild and cultivated chrysanthemums are used in herbal medicine. The wild plant is more potent. It is said to improve vision, lower fever, drive away microbes, and detoxify the body. Recent studies in Japan suggest that drinking chrysanthemum tea can lower blood pressure and help relieve headaches, dizziness, and insomnia. A chrysanthemum flower decoction also showed success in cases of angina pectoris. There are also many documented cases of this plant's ability to treat skin disorders. All of these medicinal uses have now been well documented in recent Japanese and Chinese scientific journals.

KAMPO: The flower heads are used. (*Chrysanthemi Flos*)

Main constituents: Essential oils: borneol. Other: adenine, cholin, betain, pigment.

Usage according to Japanese classics: Used to treat eye diseases. Stops cloudy vision and may be used as an eyewash. (*Ippondo-Yakusen*)

Used in Kampo prescriptions:
Choto-San.

桂 皮

CINNAMON

Lauraceae, *Cinnamomum* cassia BL.
Common name: Cinnamon
Japanese pronunciation: Keihi

Background: Recent studies indicate that cinnamon contains a substance that kills fungi, bacteria, and other microorganisms, including the one that causes botulism, and another that causes a staph infection. Cinnamon is a heady spice, too, and is used in the cuisine of East India, Morocco, Indonesia, Arabia, Mexico, Hungary, China, Greece, and many other countries around the world.

KAMPO: The bark is used (*Cinnamomi Cortex*)

Main constituents: Essential oils: cinnamic aldehyde, o-methoxy, cinnamic aldehyde, cinnamyl acetate, phenylpropyl acetate. Diterpenoides: repeated, cinncassiol A, 19-glucoside, cinnzeylanol, cinnzeylanin. Sugars: D-glucose, D-fructose, sucrose. Other: tannin.

Usage according to Japanese classics: Used mainly to treat symptoms of rising in the body (rising of the ch'i—headrushes, etc.). Also to treat severe tachycardia attacks, headaches, fever, light chills, and pain in the body with perspiration. (*Yakucho*)

Used in Kampo prescriptions:
Anchu-San, Irei-To, Inchin-Gorei-San, Unkei-To, Ogi-Kenchu-To, Oren-To,

Kakkon-To, Kakkon-To-Ka-Senkyu-Shin'i, Keishi-To, Keishi-Ka-Shakuyaku-To, Keishi-Ka-Shakuyaku-Daio-To, Keishi-Ka-Jutsubu-To, Keishi-Ka-Ryukotsu-Borei-To, Keishi-Ninjin-To, Keishi-Bukuryo-Gan, Keishi-Bukuryo-Gan-Ka-Yokuinin, Gosha-Jinki-Gan, Goshaku-San, Gorei-San, Saiko-Keishi-To, Saiko-Keishi-Kankyo-To, Saiko-Ka-Ryukotsu-Borei-To, Sairei-To, Sha-Kanzo-To, Juzen-Taiho-To, Sho-Kenchu-To, Sho-Seiryu-To, Ji-Daboku-Ippo, Tokaku-Joki-To, Toki-To, Toki-Kenchu-To, Toki-Shigyaku-Ka-Goshyuyu-Shokyo-To, Nyoshin-San, Ninjin-Yoei-To, Hachimi-Jio-Gan, Mao-To, Moku-Boi-To, Yokuinin-To, Ryo-Kei-Jutsu-Kan-To.

威霊仙

CHINESE CLEMATIS

Ranunculaceae, *Clematio chinensis* OSBECK.
Common name: Chinese clematis
Japanese pronunciation: Ireisen

Background: The sap of all plants in this family are poisonous. They are recognizable by their splayed leaves and bright yellow flowers. (The buttercup is one.)

KAMPO: The roots are used. (*Clematidis Radix*)

Main constituents: Saponins, sugars, and phenol compounds.

Used in Kampo prescriptions:
Sokei-Kakketsu-To, Kijutsu-To.

丁 子

CLOVES

Myrtaceae, *Syzygium aromaticum* MERR et PERRY.
Common name: Cloves
Japanese pronunciation: Chōji

Background: Cloves have been popular in folk medicine for centuries because of their antiseptic and pain-relieving qualities. Generations of dentists have prescribed clove oil to relieve toothaches. The herbal literature of many lands lists clove tea as a cure for nausea and to rid the stomach and intestines of gas. The Chinese use oil of clove to treat diarrhea and hernia. It is also effective against fungi such as the one that causes athlete's foot. During the Han Dynasty in China (207 B.C.–220 A.D.) court visitors were required to hold cloves in their mouth when addressing the emperor.

The tree is a handsome pyramidal evergreen with smooth, shiny leaves dotted with glands that emit the characteristically aromatic fragrance. The dried buds of the flowers are the cloves known to pharmacists and gourmet chefs around the world.

KAMPO: The flower buds are used. (*Caryophylli Flox*)

Main constituents: Essential oils: eugenol, acetyleugenol, vanillin, humulene, caryophyllene. Flavonoids: rhamnetin, kaempferol. Triterpenes: oleanolic acid. Other: tannin, fatty oils.

Pharmacological properties: Sedative, uterine contracting, antibacterial, antiviral.

Usage according to Japanese classics: Relieves hiccoughs, severe and persistent vomiting, and relieves toothache. (*Ippondo-Yakusen*)

Used in Kampo prescriptions:
Nyoshin-San, Ji-Daboku-Ippo.

黄 連

COPTIS

Ranunculaceae, *Coptis japonica* Makino
Common name: Coptis; golden thread; cankerroot.
Japanese pronunciation: Ōren

Background: The shallow root system of this plant looks like a mass of golden threads, hence the common name. It is worth its weight in gold to heavy smokers and drinkers. Early settlers in America used it for "smoker's mouth" and sore throats. In a decoction it was used to eliminate the craving for alcohol long before Alcoholics Anonymous! The plant is also used as a rural remedy for inflammation of the mucous membranes of the eye and as an anesthetic spread on the gums of teething infants. Mixed with boric acid, folk healers claim it makes a soothing eyewash.

KAMPO: The root is used. (*Coptidis Rhizoma*)

Main constituents: Alkaloids: berberine, coptisine, worenine, jateorrhizine, palmatine, magnoflorine. Other: ferulic acid, chlorogenic acid.

Pharmacological properties: Tranquilizer, anti-convulsive, stomatic, anti-diarrheal, anti-bacterial, anti-peptic ulcer, hypotensive, anti-arteriosclerosis, anti-inflammatory, immuno-moderating.

Usage according to Japanese classics: Used mainly to treat pain, discomfort, and palpitations in the chest. Also effective for discomfort in the epigastrium; for vomiting, diarrhea, and abdominal pain. (*Yakucho*)

Used in Kampo prescriptions:
Irei-To, Unsei-In, Oren-To, Oren-Gedoku-To, Keigai-Rengyo-To, Saikan-To, Saiko-Seikan-To, San'o-Shashin-To, Sei-Jo-Bofu-To, Chikujo-Untan-To, Nyoshin-San, Hange-Shashin-To.

黄　柏

CORK TREE

Rutaceae, *Phellodendron amurense* RUPR.

Common name: Amur Cork-tree; Siberian cork-tree.
Japanese pronunciation: Ōbaku

Background: The Chinese have used the bark of this tree since ancient times to treat severe fever.

KAMPO: The inner bark is peeled and used, (*Phellodendri Cortex*)

Main constituents: Alkaloids: berberine, palmatine, magnoflorine, phellodendrine, jateorrhizine. Bitter constituents: obakunone, abakulactone (Limonin). Steroids: β-sitosterol, campesterol.

Pharmacological properties: Central nervous system depressant, anti-convulsive, stomatic and anti-peptic ulcer, anti-bacterial, anti-diarrhea, hypotensive, anti-inflammatory, inhibits cyclic AMP.

Usage according to Japanese classics: It is anthelmintic and is used to treat inflammation of the digestive system, diarrhea accompanied by fever, hotness of the eyes due to febrile diseases, and fever accompanied by blood congestion. (*Ippondo-Yakusen*)

Used in Kampo prescriptions:
Unsei-In, Oren-Gedoku-To, Keigai-Rengyo-To, Saiko-Seikan-To, Jiin-Koka-To, Shichimotsu-Koka-To, Seisho-Ekki-To, Hange-Byakujutsu-Temma-To.

山茱萸

(ASIATIC) CORNELIAN CHERRY

Cornaceae, *Cornus officinalis* SIEB. et ZUCC.
Common name: Asiatic Cornelian Cherry; Dogwood
Japanese pronunciation: Sanshuyu

Background: This is the dogwood of the Far East with an affinity for the liver and kidneys. In China, the fruit has been used for kidney deficiency, impotence, lumbago, vertigo, incontinence, and blurry vision. In the U.S. Civil War dogwood bark was used by the South as a substitute for quinine during the blockade of its ports by the North.

KAMPO: The fruit is used with the seeds removed. (*Corni furctus*)

Main constituents: monoterpene glycosides: morronside, loganin, sweroside. Triterpenoids: ursolic acid. Saponin: cornin. Tannins: tellimagrandin I, II, isoterchebin, cornusiin A, B. Organic acids: tartaric acid, malic acid, gallic acid. Others: oleanolic acid.

Pharmacological properties: Anti-diabetic, anti-allergic, immunomoderating.

Usage according to Japanese classics: Warms the spleen and stomach; warms the knees and lower back; relieves pain and paralysis caused by damp and cold; aids urinary tract function; stops geriatric polyuria, tinnitus, and headaches. (*Koho-Yakugi*)

Used in Kampo prescriptions:
Gosha-Jinki-Gan, Hachimi-Jio-Gan,
Rokumi-Gan.

延胡索

CORYDALIS

Papaveraceae, *Corydalis turtschaninouli* Bess. f. yanhusuo Y.H. chan et C.C. Hsu
Common name: Corydalis
Japanese pronunciation: Engosaku

Background: This is a powerful plant, the source of the alkaloid bulbocariine which was used in orthodox medicines to treat convulsions, Parkinson's disease and Meniere's disease. In Chinese traditional medicine, corydalis is a major pain reliever used for menstrual cramps, gastric and abdominal pain, and headaches.

Caution: This is another dangerous herb that should be used only by trained herbalists.
KAMPO: The tuber is used. (*Cordalis Tuber*)

Main constituents: Alkaloids: *l*-corydaline, dehydrocorydaline, bulbocapnine, coptisine, protopine, *l*-tatrahydropalmatine. Other: palmitic acid, oleic acid, linoleic acid, stigmasterol.

Pharmacological properties: Useful for its sedative, analgesic, antispasmodic, and anti-peptic ulcer actions.

Usage according to Japanese classics: Used for treating pain in the chest, lower abdomen, and various other parts of the body. (*Ippondo-Yakusen*)

Used in Kampo prescriptions:
Anchu-San.

木 香

COSTUS

Compositae, *Saussurea lappa* CLARKE.
Common name: Costus
Japanese pronunciation: Mokkō

Background: The fragrant root of this annual herb native to Kashmir yields a volatile oil commonly used in perfumery and for preserving furs. This versatile plant can also be used to treat a wide variety of illnesses.

KAMPO: The root is used for healing. (*Saussureae Radix*)

Main constituents: Essential oils: Saussurealacone, costuslactone, β-elemen. Alkaloids: saussurine. Other: tannins, bitter constituents.

Pharmacological properties: Central nervous system suppressant, smooth muscle relaxant, antibacterial.

Usage according to Japanese classics: Used to treat severe vomiting and diarrhea due to bad foodstuffs, and diarrhea due to infectious diseases. Also aids digestion and helps insure safe pregnancy. Relieves chest pain, abdominal pain, discomfort of the epigastrium, and hard stagnation in the abdomen. Aids stomach function and increases the appetite. (*Ippondo-Yakusen*)

Used in Kampo prescriptions:
Kihi-To, Kami-Kihi-To, Jinso-In,
Nyoshin-San.

麻 黄

EPHEDRA

Ephedraceae, *Ephedra sinica* STAPF.
Common name: Ephedra

Japanese pronunciation: Maō

Background: This herb has been used as a decongestant in the Orient for 3,000 years. Researchers finally isolated the key ingredient, ephedrine, in the laboratory. However, the isolated drug raised blood pressure markedly, and is now seldom used in treating asthma. Herbalists, however, use the whole plant which contains six other related alkaloids. One of them, pseudoephedrine, actually reduces the heart rate and lowers blood pressure. In China, the herb is also used to treat arthritis and flu. NOTE: The herb should be avoided in patients with hypertension, glaucoma, hyperthyroidism, prostate enlargement, and coronary thrombosis, It should not be taken by anyone using MAOI anti-depressant.

KAMPO: The stems of this plant are used, (*Ephedrae Herba*)

Main constituents: Alkaloids: *l*-ephedrine, i-N-methlephedrine, δ-pseudoephedrine, ephedradine A, B, C. Flavonoids: feruloyl histamine.

Pharmacological properties: Stimulates the central nervous system and sympathetic nervous system, hypotensive, antitussive, sudorific, cholygogous, anti-inflammatory, anti-allergic, inhibits production of prostaglandin, BUN reducing.

Usage according to Japanese classics: Used mainly to treat asthma-like respiratory disorders, coughing, and edema. Also for severe and light chills, lack of perspiration, general body pain, joint pain, and yellow general edema. (*Yakucho*)

Used in Kampo prescriptions:
Eppi-Ka-Jutsu-To, Kakkon-To, Kakkon-To-Ka-Senkyu-Sehin'i, Goko-To, Goshaku-San, Sho-Seiryu-To, Shimpi-To, Bofu-Tsusho-San, Mao-To, Mao-Bushi-Saishin-To, Ma-Kyo-Kan-Seki-To, Ma-Kyo-Yoku-Kan-To, Yokuinin-To.

呉茱萸

EVODIA

Rutaceae, *Evodia rutaecarpa* BENTH. or E. officinalis DODE.
Common name: Evodia
Japanese pronunciation: Goshuyu

Background: Long ago, in Japan, China, and India this herb won renown as a highly effective anthelmintic against pin worms and as a tonic for the uterus.

KAMPO: The fruit is used. (*Evodiae Fructus*)

Main constituents: Alkaloids: evodiamine, hydroxyevodiamine, rutaecarpine, synephrine. Essential oils: evodene, limonin. Other: cyclic GMP.

Pharmacological properties: Analgesic and interferon inducing.

Usage according to Japanese classics: Used mainly to treat nausea and vomiting accompanied by a bloated feeling in the abdomen. (*Yakucho*)

Used in Kampo prescriptions:
Unkei-To, Goshuyu-To, Toki-Shigyaku-Ka-Goshyuyu-Sho-To.

茴 香

FENNEL

Umbelliferae, *Foeniculum vulgare* MILL.
Common name: Fennel
Japanese pronunciation: Uikyo

Background: All parts of the fennel plant are safe for human consumption and work well as a spice or vegetable. In medieval times fennel was one of nine sacred herbs with the power to cure the nine basic causes of disease. The famous battle of Marathon, 490 B.C., was fought on a field of fennel. Throughout history, fennel has been used to break up kidney stones, prevent nausea and gout, clear the liver and lungs, promote the flow of breast milk, and serve as an eyewash.

KAMPO: The fruit is used. (*Foeniculi Frunctus*)

Main constituents: Essential oils: anethole, estragole, limonene, anisadehyde, α-pinene. Other: fatty oils.

Pharmacological properties: Stimulates the digestive function. Used as carminative, diuretic, and stimulant.

Usage according to Japanese classics: Used as an appetite suppressant. Fennel tea is also used to sooth the stomach.

Used in Kampo prescriptions:
Anchu-San.

防 風

FERN

Umbelliferae, *Ledebouriella seseloides* WOLF. (f).
Common name: Fern
Japanese pronunciation: Bōfu

Background: Because St. Patrick put a curse on ferns they have no flowers, says an old Irish legend. The saint's anger may have been aroused by the fact that ferns are associated in folklore with serpents. Old-time folk healers believed that any plant that was a "snake plant" was powerful medicine.

KAMPO: The root of the fern is used. (*Ledebouriellae Radix*)

Main constituents: Procoumarins: deltoin, bergapten, psoraien. Cromons: hamaudol. Others: cimifugin, 5-o-methylvisamminol.

Pharmacological properties: Anti-inflammatory.

Usage according to Japanese classics: Used to relieve painful, numb joints; migraine headaches; red, blood-congested eyes; spasms in the extremities; painful and stiff back and neck muscles; and inability to turn the head. (*Ippondo-Yakusen*)

Used in Kampo prescriptions:
Keigai-Rengyo-To, Jumi-Haidoku-To, Shofu-San, Senkyu-Chacho-San, Sokei-Kakketsu-To, Dai-Bofu-To, Ji-Zuso-Ippo, Choto-San, Toki-Inshi, Bofu-Tsusho-San, Rikko-San.

羌 活

NOTCHED LEAF FERN

Umbelliferae, *Notopterygium forbesii* BOISS.

Common name: Notched Leaf Fern
Japanese pronunciation: Kyokatsu

KAMPO: The rhizome of this fern is used. (*Notopterygii Rhizoma*)

Main constituents: Essential oils: limonene, pinene, coumarin derivatives, arginine.

Pharmacological properties: Interferon inducing.

Usage according to Japanese classics: Used for illness where there is numbness, chill, and pain caused by wind, cold, or dampness. Relieves pain and stiffness in the joints and muscles, also various eye diseases, painful and inflamed eyes, cloudy vision, swollen joints, numbness, itchy skin, and spasms. (*Ippondo, Yakusen*)

Used in Kampo prescriptions:
Senkyu-Chacho-San, Sokei-Kakketsu-To, Dai-Bofu-To.

連 翹

FORSYTHIA

Oleaceae, *Forsythia suspensa* VAHL. *F. viridissima* LINDL. or *F. koreana* NAKAI.
Common name: Forsythia, Weeping Golden Bell
Japanese pronunciation: Rengyō

Background: The ancient masters used this handsome plant as an antipyretic, antidote, and antiphlogistic. It was considered effective in treating heat rash, swelling of the lymph glands, erysipelas, and breast tumors.

KAMPO: The fruit is used in Kampo. (*Forsythiae Fructus*)

Main constituents: Triterpenoids: betulinic acid, ursolic acid, oleanolic acid. Lignin and glycosides: phillygenin, δ-pinoresinol, phillyrin, arctiin. Flavonoids: rutin.

Pharmacological properties: Anti-bacterial, anti-allergic.

Usage according to Japanese classics: Used to treat scabies, pimples, and other purulent skin diseases. (*Ippondo-Yakusen*)

Used in Kampo prescriptions:
Keigai-Rengyo-To, Saiko-Seikan-To, Sei-Jo-Bofu-To, Ji-Zuso-Ippo, Bofu-Tsusho-San.

地 黄

CHINESE FOXGLOVE

Scrophulariaceae, *Rehmannia glutinosa* LIB., var, *purpurea* MAK.
Common name: Chinese foxglove
Japanese pronunciation: Jiō

Background: Foxglove is among the loveliest, most important, and most dangerous of all medicinal plants. Its long green leaves are powdered into digitalis, the heart stimulant that keeps millions of patients alive. Yet it is a deadly poison, as likely to stop a heart as keep it going. The root of the Oriental plant is used in Japan and China as a tonic for the blood, and to help diabetics. The plant has an affinity for the liver and kidneys as well as for the heart.

KAMPO: The root is used. (*Rehmanniae Radix*)

Main constituents: Glycosides: catapol, aucubin. Sterols: β-sitosterol. Sugars: D-glucose, D-galactose, D-fructose, sucrose, raffinose, stachyose. Other: arginine, mannitol.

Pharmacological properties: Hypoglycemic, anti-coagulant, diuretic, mild laxative.

Usage according to Japanese classics: Used mainly to treat various conditions related to the blood (blood stagnation) and fluid metabolism. (*Yakucho*)

Used in Kampo prescriptions:
Unsei-In, Kyuki-Kyogai-To, Keigai-Rengyo-To, Gosha-Jinki-Gan, Gorin-San, Saiko-Seikan-To, Sammotsu-Ogon-To, Jiin-Koka-To, Shichimotsu-Koka-To, Shimotsu-To, Sha-Kanzo-To, Juzen-Taiho-To, Juncho-To, Shofu-San, Sokei-Kakketsu-To, Dai-Bofu-To, Chorei-To-Go-Shimotsu-To, Toki-Inshi, Ninjin-Yoei-To, Hachimi-Jio-Gan, Ryutan-Shakan-To, Rokumi-Gan.

良 姜

GALANGA

Zingiberaceae, *Alpina officinarum* HANCE.
Common name: Galanga
Japanese pronunciation: Ryōkyō

KAMPO: The rhizome of this plant is used. (*Alpiniae Officinarum Rhizoma*)

Main constituents: Essential oils: 1, 8-cineol, methylcinnamate, eugenol, pinene, cadinene. Flavonoids: galangin, kaempferol, kaempferide. Pungent constituents: galangol. Other: starch, tannin.

Pharmacological properties: Inhibits the production of prostaglandin.

Usage according to Japanese classics: Used to treat coldness of the stomach and abdominal pain. Aids digestion. (*Ippondo-Yakusen*)

Used in Kampo prescriptions:
Anchu-San.

釣藤鈎

GAMBIR VINE

Rubiaceae, *Uncaria rhunchopylla* MIQ. or U. *sinesis* OLIV.
Common name: Gambir vine
Japanese pronunciation: Chōtokō

Background. This is a woody vine with bright yellow flowers found in abundance in the tropics.

KAMPO: The hooklike joints of this plant are used. (*Uncariae Ramulus et Uncus*)

Main constituents: Alkaloids: rynchophylline, isorhynchopophylline, cornynoxeine, hirsutine, 3-α-dihydrocadambine, 3-β-isodihydrocadambine.

Pharmacological properties: Hypotensive.

Used in Kampo prescriptions:
Shichimotsu-Koka-To, Choto-San, Yoku-Kan-San, Yoku-Kan-San-Ka-Chimpi-Hange.

阿仙薬

GAMBIR LEAVES

Rubiaceae, *Uncaria gambir* ROXB.
Common name: Catechu, gambir
Japanese pronunciation: Asenyaku

KAMPO: The leaves and young twigs are used. (*Gambir*)

Main constituents: Catechins: catechin, d-epicatechin, quercetin. Flavonoids: chalcone-flavan dimer. Alkaloids: gambirtannin, dihydrogambirtannin.

Pharmacological properties: Stops thirst.

山梔子

GARDENIA

Rubiaceae, *Gardenia jasminoides* Ellis.
Common name: Gardenia
Japanese pronunciation: Sanshishi

Background: Gardenias are a favorite folk remedy throughout the Far East. A paste of the plant mixed with flour and wine is used as a poultice on twists, sprains, bruises, and abcesses. Villagers swear it is highly effective in cases of injury to tendons, ligaments, joints, and muscles.

KAMPO: The fruit of this plant is used in Kampo. (*Gardeniae Fructus*)

Main constituents: Glycosides: geniposide, genipin, gentiobioside, gardenoside. Yellow pigment: crocin, crocetin. Flavonoids: gardenin. Other: fatty oils (14–18% in the fruit), mannitol, β-sitosterol.

Pharmacological properties: Analgesic, laxative, suppresses the secretion of stomach juices, cholagogous, hepatoprotective, hypotensive, anti-arteriosclerosis, anticoagulant.

Usage according to Japanese classics: Used mainly to treat pain and discomfort in the chest. Also to treat jaundice. (*Yakucho*)

Used in Kampo prescriptions:
Inchinko-To, Unsei-In, Oren-Gedoku-To, Kami-Kihi-To, Kami-Shoyo-San, Keigai-Rengyo-To, Gorin-San, Saiko-Seikan-To, Shin'i-Seihai-To, Sei-Jo-Bofu-To, Seihai-To, Bofu-Tsusho-San, Ryutan-Shakan-To.

竜 胆

CHINESE GENTIAN

Gentianaceae, *Gentiana scabra* Bge.
Common name: Chinese Gentian
Japanese pronunciation: Ryutan

Background: Greeks, Egyptians and Arabs all used gentian in cures for stomach and liver ailments, as a tonic, and to ward off pestilence. It has also been used to raise white blood cell counts. Pregnant woman or anyone with high blood pressure is advised not to take gentian root.

KAMPO: The root of this plant is used. (*Gentianae Scabrae Radix*)

Main constituents: Bitter constituents: monoperpone glycosides, gentiopicroside, trifloraside, swertiamarin. Kisantone derivatives: gentisin. Sugars: gentianose, sucrose.

Pharmacological properties: Anti-allergic.

Usage according to Japanese classics: Used to relieve a feeling of fever in the bones and joints due to venereal diseases, and inflammation with blood congestion of the eyes. (*Ippondo-Yakusen*)

Used in Kampo prescriptions:
Sokei-Kakketsu-To, Rikko-San,
Ryutan-Shakan-To.

細辛

CHINESE WILD GINGER

Artistolochiaceae, *Asiasarum sieboldi* F. MAEKAWA or *Asiasarum heterotropoides* F. MAEKAWA var. *mandshuricum* F. MAEKAWA.
Common name: Chinese Wild Ginger
Japanese pronunciation: Saishin

Background: Ginger is spicy to the tongue and soothing to the digestive system. Cooks in the Orient rarely stir-fry vegetables without first browning a piece of the fresh root.

In Japan, a ginger-oil massage is a traditional treatment for spinal and joint problems. Other herbalists recommend hot ginger compresses and baths to relieve gout, arthritis, headaches and spinal pain. Ginger compresses are used in many countries worldwide to relieve sinus congestion, kidney problems, menstrual cramps, and various other aches and pains. A piece of cotton soaked in ginger is a common treatment for earache. Modern medicine recognizes many of ginger's time-honored virtues. It is known to stimulate the flow of blood to a given area, rid the stomach of gas, and to aid in the digestion of fatty foods. Recent research also supports the notion that ginger prevents motion sickness and morning sickness.

KAMPO: The whole root of this plant is used. (*Asiasari Radix*)

Main constituents: Essential oils: β-pinene, 1, 8-cineol, safrole, methyleugenol. Alkaloids: higenamine. Lignin: i-asarinin.

Pharmacological properties: Antipyretic: analgesic, anti-allergic, inhibits cyclic AMP.

Usage according to Japanese classics: Used mainly to treat conditions in which the pathogen is stagnant in the chest and diaphragm; also to treat fluid irregularities. (*Yakucho*)

Used in Kampo prescriptions:
Sho-Seiryu-To, Toki-Shigyaku-Ka-Goshuyu-Shokyo-To, Mao-Bushi-Saishin-To, Rikko-San, Ryo-Kan-Kyo-Mi-Shin-Ge-Nin-To.

山 椒

PEPPER

Rutaceae, *Zanthoxylum piperitum DC.*
Common name: Japanese pepper, Szechuan pepper
Japanese pronunciation: Sanshō

Background: In Chinese medicine, hot pepper has been traditionally used to increase appetite and to treat arthritis and rheumatism. Pepper is popular in folk medicine, used to treat abdominal pain, vomiting, diarrhea, chilblains, ringworm, malaria, bruises and hematomas.

KAMPO: The ripe fruit is used. (*Zanthoxyli Fructus*)

Main constituents: Essential oils: *dl*-limonene, citronellal. Pungent constituents: sanshool, sanshoamide. Other: xanthoxylin, xanthoxin, tannin.

Pharmacological properties: Anti-tumor, inhibits cyclic AMP.

Usage according to Japanese classics: Relieves coldness and pain in the abdomen; kills intestinal parasites; warms the spleen and stomach; and disperses cold. (*Ippondo-Yakusen*)

Used in Kampo prescriptions:
Dai-Kenchu-To, Toki-To.

生 姜

GINGER

Zingiberaceae, *Zingiber officinale* Rosc.
Common name: Ginger

Japanese pronunciation: Shokyō

Background: (See Chinese Wild Ginger.)

KAMPO: The rhizome of this plant is used. (*Zingiberis Rhizoma*)

Main constituents: Essential oils: zingiberen. Pungent constituents: gingerol, zingerone, shogaol.

Pharmacological properties: Central nervous system suppresant, antipyretic, anti-convulsive, antitussive, antiemitic. Promotes the secretion of saliva, anti-peptic ulcer, stimulates peristalsis, inhibits the production of prostaglandin, cardiotonic.

Usage according to Japanese classics: Used mainly to treat the imbalance and stagnation of fluids in the body. Also to treat vomiting, coughing, diarrhea, cold extremities, discomfort and unsettledness, pain in the abdomen, chest, and lower back. (*Yakucho*)

Used in Kampo prescriptions:
Oren-To, Keishi-Ninjin-To, Saiko-Keishi-Kankyo-To, Sho-Seiryu-To, Dai-Kenchu-To, Dai-Bofu-To, Toki-To, Ninjin-To, Hange-Shashin-To, Hange-Byakujutsu-Temma-To, Ryo-Kan-Kyo-Mi-Shin-Ge-Nin-To, Ryo-Kyo-Jutsu-Kan-To.

(The cork skin of the root is removed in the following Kampo prescriptions: Saiko-Keishi-Kankyo-To, Shoseiryu-To, Hange-Shashin-To, Ryo-Kyo-Jutsu-kan-To.)

人 参

GINSENG

Araliaceae, *Panax ginseng* C.A. MAY.
Common name: Ginseng
Japanese pronunciation: Ninjin

Background: This herb has been touted as the "king of tonics," a prolonger of life and cure for all human ills for thousands of years—not to mention the cornerstone of a multimillion-dollar ginseng trade. Ginseng madness was once so strong that people would kill to acquire the root. Perhaps the fever may strike again, as it is now touted as a cure for the stress of modern life. Olympic athletes take it as a way to enhance their powers of endurance. What do laboratory tests show?

Ginseng may indeed, actually slow down the effects of aging, protect cells from radiation damage, and moderate the effects of a high-cholesterol diet. Manchurian ginseng is the most potent but is very, very expensive. Korean is the best substitute.

KAMPO: The root of the Korean ginseng is used. (*Ginseng Radix*)

Main constituents: Saponins: ginsenoside Ro, Ra, Rb_1, Rb_2, Rb_3, Rc, Rd, Re, Rf, Rg_1, Rg_2, Rh, 20-glucoginsenoside Rf. Essential oils: panaxynol, β-elemene. Fat soluble constituents: β-sitosterol, glucoside. Sugars: D-glucose, D-fructose, sucrose, maltose, trisaccharide A, B, C. Other: amino acid, peptide, choline, vitamin B complex, ATP, arginine, etc.

Pharmacological properties: Stimulates the central nervous system. In varying dosage suppresses the central nervous system; speeds up recovery from fatigue. Anti-stress, tonic; increases male hormones; increases the synthesis of proteins, DNA and fats, speeds up recovery from radiation exposure, hypotensive, improves heart circulation, hypoglycemic, improves fat metabolism, anticoatulant, increases cholesteron secretion, anti-gastric ulcer, improves malaise from dialysis, immuno-stimulating, increases cell life.

Usage according to Japanese classics: Aids in recovery from general functional upset of the body, expels various pathogens. Stops severe thirst and general discomfort; stops vomiting due to unhygenic food; stops diarrhea, cold in the extremities, shortness of breath rapid breathing, shallow breathing, abdominal pain, spontaneous perspiration. Supplements body fluids and stops mental anxiety and heart palpitations. Relieves malaria-like acute febrile diseases. Aids the digestive function and protects good ch'i. Is used for hemorrhaging and postpartum fatigue. Expels internal purulence. Is used for various acute diseases, fatigue, and weakness. (*Ippondo-Yakusen*)

Used in Kampo prescriptions:
Unkei-To, Oren-To, Kami-Kihi-To, Kihi-To, Keishi-Ninjin-To, Keihi-To, Goshuyu-To, Saikan-To, Saiko-Ka-Ryukotsu-Borei-To, Saiko-Keishi-To, Saiboku-To, Sairei-To, Sha-Kanzo-To, Juzen-Taiho-To, Sho-Saiko-To-Ka-Kikyo-Sekko, Jinso-In, Seisho-Ekki-To, Seishin-Renshi-In, Dai-Kenchu-To, Dai-Bofu-To, Chikujo-Untan-To, Choto-San, Toki-To, Nyoshin-San, Ninjin-To, Ninjin-Yoei-To, Baku-mondo-To, Hange-Shashin-To, Hange-Byakujutsu-Temma-To, Byakko-Ka-Ninjin-To, Bukuryuo-In, Bukuryo-In-Go-Hange-Koboku-To, Hochu-Ekki-To, Moku-Boi-To, Rikkunshi-To.

山楂子

HAWTHORN

Rosaceae, *Crataegus cuneata* Sieb. Et Zucc.
Common name: Crataegus, Chinese hawthorn
Japanese pronunciation: Sanzashi

Background: The Chinese recommend this plant to improve digestion. It also dilates the blood vessels to lower blood pressure and dissolves cholesterol deposits in the lining of the blood vessels.

KAMPO: The fruits are used. (*Crataegi Fructus*)

Main constituents: Flavonoids: quercetin. Saponin: ursolic acid, oleanolic acid, crataegolic acid. Digestive enzymes: protease, amylase. Other: abundant amount of vitamin C.

Pharmacological properties: Accelerates alcoholic metabolism.

Usage according to Japanese classics: Used to treat digestive problems due to the eating of meat.

Used in Kampo prescription:
Keihi-To.

薏苡仁

JOB'S TEARS

Gramineae, *Coix lachryma-jobi* L. var. *ma-yuen* Stapf.
Common name: Job's tears, Coix
Japanese pronunciation: Yokui'nin

Background: This plant is a common food item in China and Japan and contains 17% protein. A liquor fermented from the seeds is often used to relieve rheumatic pains.

KAMPO: The seeds of this plant are used. (*Coicia Semen*)

Main constituents: Acid components: glycoside of 3, 4-dihydroxybenzaldehyde, etc. Triterpenoids: fredelin, isoarborinol, etc. Essential oils: palmitic acid, myristic acid, etc. Others: starches, proteins, β-sitosterol, coixenolide, amino acids, RNase, vitamin B_1, etc.

Pharmacological properties: Central nervous system suppressant, muscle relaxant, anti-tumor.

Usage according to Japanese classics: Used mainly to treat tumors. (*Ippondo-Yakusen*)

Used in Kampo prescriptions:
Keishi-Bukuryo-Gan-Ka-Yokuinin,
Ma-Kyo-Yoku-Kan-To, Yokuinin-To.

大 棗

JUJUBE (Fruit)

Rhamnaceae, *Zizyphus jujuba* MILL. var. *inermis* REHD.
Common name: Jujube, Red Date, Ziziphus
Japanese pronunciation: Taiso

Background: Herbal healers throughout the Far East from China to Malaysia are familiar with this herb. Traditionally, it is considered to have an affinity for the heart, spleen, liver and gall bladder. It is used as a sedative to the liver, a cardiotonic, and to treat insomnia and cold sweats.

KAMPO: The fruit is used (*Zizyphi Fructus*)

Main constituents: Triterpine: oleanolic acid, butulinic acid, alphitolic acid and p-croumaric esters, ursolic acid. Saponins: zizyphus saponin. Others: sugars, malic acid, tartaric acid, cyclic AMP, cyclic GMP.

Pharmacological properties: Anti-allergic, anti-peptic ulcer, anti-stress.

Usage according to Japanese classics: Used mainly to treat severe cramps. Also relieves coughing, severe palpitations that seem to rise upward in the body, discomfort, pain and abdominal pain. (*Yakucho*)

Used in Kampo prescriptions:
Irei-To, Eppi-Ka-Jutsu-To, Ogi-Kenchu-To, Oren-To, Kakkon-To, Kakkon-To-Ka-Senkyu-Shin'i, Kam-Baku-Taiso-To, Kihi-To, Kami-Kihi-To, Keishi-Ka-Shakuyaku-To, Keishi-Ka-Shakuyaku-Daio-To, Keishi-Ka-Jutsu-Bu-To, Keishi-To, Goshuyu-To, Goshaku-San, Saikan-To, Saiko-Ka-Ryukotsu-Borei-To, Saiko-Keishi-To, Saiboku-To, Sairei-To, Shikunshi-To, Sha-Kanzo-To, Sho-Kenchu-To, Sho-Saiko-To, Sho-Saiko-To-Ka-Kikyo-Sekko, Jinso-In, Seihai-To, Dai-Saiko-To, Toki-Kenchu-To, Toki-Shigyaku-Ka-Goshuyu-Shokyo-To, Haino-San-Kyu-To, Bakumondo-To, Hange-Shashin-To, Heii-San, Boi-Ogi-To. Hochu-Ekki-To, Rikkunshi-To.

酸棗仁

JUJUBE (Seed)

Rhamnaceae, *zizyphus jujuba* MILL. (Z. *Vulgaris* LAM. var. *spinosus* BGE.)
Common name: Jujube date, Zizyphus
Japanese pronunciation: Sansōnin

Background: The Chinese jujube date is used in a wide variety of herbal formulas and is found in dried form in most Oriental markets. Families use it to add zest to soups and stews. It gives energy to the body, relieves nervous exhaustion, insomnia, apprehension, forgetfulness, dizziness, and clamminess.

KAMPO: The seeds of this plant are used. (*Zizyphi Spinosi Semen*)

Main constituents: Fatty acids: palmitic acid, stearic acid, oleic acid, linolenic acid, etc. Sterols: β-sitosterol, etc. Saponin: jujuboside A, B, C, etc.

Pharmacological properties: Central nervous system suppressant, anti-stress.

Usage according to Japanese classics: Mainly used to treat congestion of chest and diaphragm area, and insomnia. (*Yakucho*)

Used in Kampo prescriptions:
Kami-Kihi-To, Kihi-To, Sansonin-To.

葛 根

KUDZU

Leguminosae, *Pueraria lobata* OHWI or P. *lobata* OHWI var. *chinensislobata*
Common name: Kudzu
Japanese pronunciation: Kakkon

Background: Kudzu is common in the Far East. The Chinese have used it for centuries to relax tight, painful muscles in the neck, shoulders, and back.

KAMPO: The root is used with the outer skin removed. (*Puerariae Radix*)

Main constituents: Flavonoids: dadzein, daidzin, puerarin, genistein, formononetin, puerarol, kakkonein. Other: starch, D-mannitol, miroestrol, succinic acid, allantoin.

Pharmacological properties: Anti-spasmodic, antipyretic, stimulates peristalsis, affects the circulatory system (hypotensive, increases blood flow in the brain, aorta, etc.).

Usage according to Japanese classics: Used mainly to treat stiffness in the neck and back. Also used to treat breathing difficulties when perspiration is present. (*Yakucho*)

Used in Kampo prescriptions:
Kakkon-To, Kakkon-To-Ka-Senkyu-Shin'i, Shoma-Kakkon-To, Jinso-In.

麦門冬

LILY

Liliaceae, *Ophiopogon japonicus* KER-GAWL.
Common name: Japanese Lily
Japanese pronunciation: Bakumondō

Background: The lily has one high honor in history. In the 8th century, the Emperor Charlemagne ordered a group of healing herbs to be planted throughout the kingdom, the Holy Roman Empire. The lily was one of the herbs chosen by this monarch.

KAMPO: The root of this plant is used. (*Ophiopogonis Tuber*)

Main constituents: Steroid-saponins: opiopogonin A-D. Monoisoflavonoids: ophiopogonone A, B. Other: β-sitosterol, sugars.

Pharmacological properties: Hypoglycemic, anti-inflammatory.

Usage according to Japanese classics: Used to treat coughing, and fever accompanied by discomfort; supplements the body's fluids when fever or symptoms of dryness are present. (*Ippondo-Yakusen*)

Used in Kampo prescriptions:
Unkei-To, Jiin-Koka-To, Jiin-Shiho-To, Sha-Kanzo-To, Shin'i-Seihai-To, Seisho-Ekki-To, Seishin-Renshi-In, Seihai-To, Chikujo-Untan-To, Choto-San, Bakumondo-To.

甘 草

LICORICE

Leguminosae, *Glycyrrhiza glabra* L. var. *glandulifera* REG. et HERD. G. *uralensis* FISCH.
Common name: Licorice
Japanese pronunciation: Kanzō

Background: The licorice root was mentioned in the very first Chinese herbal, thousands of years ago, and was introduced into Europe centuries later. The Blackfoot Indians used licorice to cure earaches. Other uses in various cultures include treatment of dropsy, fever, menstrual cramps, flu; hypoglycemia, and coughs. The chief component is 50 times sweeter than sugar! For a plant known primarily as a candy flavoring it has a remarkably long list of pharmacological properties.

KAMPO: The root is used in Japanese herbal medicine. (*Glycyrrhizae Radix*)

Main constituents: Saponins: glycyrrhizin. Flavonoids: liquiritin, licoricone, licoflavone, licoricidin. Other: putresoin.

Pharmacological properties: Sedative, antispasmodic, antitussive, anti-peptic ulcer, cholagogous, hepatoprotective, anti-inflammatory, anti-allergic, inhibits cyclic AMP, steroid hormone-like actions, anti-mutation.

Usage according to Japanese classics: Used mainly to treat acute symptoms. Also to treat acute abdominal cramps and pain, cold extremities, restlessness, "rising symptoms," and other acute symptoms. (*Yakucho*)

Used in Kampo prescriptions:
Anchu-San, Irei-To, Unkei-To, Eppi-Ka-Jutsu-To, Ogi-Kenchu-To, Oren-To, Otsuji-To, Kakkon-To, Kakkon-To-Ka-Senkyu-Shin'i, Kami-Kihi-To, Kami-Shoyo-San, Kam-Baku-Taiso-To, Kikyo-To, Kihi-To, Kyuki-Kyogai-To, Keigai-Rengyo-To, Keishi-Ka-Shakuyaku-To, Keishi-Ka-Shakuyaku-Daio-To, Keishi-Ka-Jutsubu-To, Keishi-Ka-Ryukotsu-Borei-To, Keishi-To, Keishi-Ninjin-To, Keihi-To, Koso-San, Goko-To, Goshaku-San, Gorin-San, Saikan-To, Saiko-Ka-Ryukotsu-Borei-To, Saiko-Keishi-To, Saiko-Keishi-Kankyo-To, Sha-Kanzo-To, Saiko-Seikan-To, Saiboku-To, Sairei-To, Sansonin-To, Jiin-Koka-To, Jiin-Shiho-To, Shigyaku-San, Shikunshi-To, Shakuyaku-Kanzo-To, Juzen-Taiho-To, Jumi-Haidoku-To, Juncho-To, Sho-Kenchu-To, Sho-Saiko-To, Saho-Saiko-To-Ka-Kikyo-Sekko, Sho-Seiryu-To, Shoma-Kakkon-To, Shofu-San, Jinso-In, Shimpi-To, Sei-Jo-Bofu-To, Seisho-Ekki-To, Seishin-Renshi-In, Seihai-To, Senkyu-Chacho-San, Sokei-Kakketsu-To, Daio-Kanzo-To, Dai-Bofu-To, Chikujo-Untan-To, Ji-Zuso-Ippo, Ji-Daboku-Ippo, Choi-Joki-To, Choto-San, Tsu-Do-San, Tokaku-Joki-To, Toki-Inshi, Toki-Kenchu-To, Toki-Shigyaku-Ka-Goshuyu-Shokyo-To, Toki-To, Nichin-To, Nijutsu-To, Nyoshin-San, Ninjin-To, Ninjin-Yoei-To, Haino-San-Kyu-To, Bakumondo-To, Hange-Shashin-To, Byakko-Ka-Ninjin-To, Heii-San, Boi-Ogi-To, Bofu-Tsusho-San, Hochu-Ekki-To, Mao-To, Ma-Kyo-Kan-Seki-To, Ma-kyo-Yoku-Kan-To, Ryo-Kan-kyo-Mi-Shin-Ge-Nin-To, Ryo-Kyo-Jutsu-Kan-To, Ryo-Kei-Jutsu-Kan-To.

連 肉

LOTUS

Nymphaeaceae, *Nelumbo nucifera* GAERTN.
Common name: Lotus
Japanese pronunciation: Renniku

Background: Every part of the lotus plant is used in herbal medicine. The stem is used to relieve congestion in the chest. The peduncle is used for stomach aches, to calm the fetus, and to treat leukorrhea. The seeds are used for insomnia, spermatorrhoea, and diarrhea. The stamens are a preventive for premature ejaculation.

KAMPO: The seeds are used in Kampo. (*Nelumbinins Semen*)

Main constituents: Alkaloids: lotusine, demethylcoclaurine, oxoushinsuine, methylcorpoalline. Other: starch, raffinose, proteins, fats.

Pharmacological properties: Relaxes the smooth muscles.

Usage according to Japanese classics: Used to treat diarrhea which has continued for a long time. (*Ippondo-Yakusen*)

Used in Kampo prescriptions:
Seishin-Renshi-In, Keihi-To.

厚 朴

MAGNOLIA (Bark)

Magnoliaceae, *Magnolia obovata* THUMB.
Common name: Magnolia
Japanese pronunciation: Kōboku

Background: Traditionally, in China, the magnolia was used as an analgesic and decongestant for ailments of the nose and for sinusitis.

KAMPO: The bark of the tree is used in Japan. (*Magnoliae Cortex*)

Main constituents: Essential oils: β-eudesmol, α-pinene, β-pinene, camphene, limonene. Alkaloids: magnocurarine, magnoflorine. Diphenols: magnolol, honokiol.

Pharmacological properties: Muscle relaxant, anti-convulsant, sedative, anti-peptic ulcer, anti-inflammatory, anti-allergic, antibacterial.

Usage according to Japanese classics: Used mainly to treat distention of the chest, and swelling and distention of the abdomen. Also to treat abdominal pain. (*Yakucho*)

Used in Kampo prescriptions:
Irei-To, Goshaku-San, Juncho-To, Saiboku-To, Shimp-To, Dai-Joki-To,

Tsu-Do-San, Toki-To, Hange-Koboku-To, Bukuryo-In-Go-Hange-Koboku-To, Heii-San, Mashinin-Gan.

辛夷

MAGNOLIA (Blossoms)

Magnoliaceae, *Magnolia salicaflora* MAXIM, M. *Kobus* DC.
Common name: Magnolia

KAMPO: The blossoms of this plant are used. (*Magnoliae Flos*)

Main constituents: Essential oils: citral cineol, α-pinene, eugenol. Alkaloids: d-coclaurine, N-methyl coclaurine, d-reticuline. Organic acids: palmitic acid, linolenic acid, vanillic acid.

Pharmacological properties: Muscle relaxant, anti-allergy.

Used in Kampo prescriptions:
Kakkon-To-Ka-Senkyu-Shin'i,
Shin'i-Seihai-To.

膠飴

MALT SUGAR

Gramineae
Common name: Malt sugar
Japanese pronunciation: Kōi

KAMPO: This is a sugar made from powdering rice, wheat and other grains, then adding the germ. (*Saccharum Granorum*)

Main constituents: maltose, dextrin, proteins, fats.

Usage according to Japanese classics: Strengthens and tones the body. Stops coughing and the secretion of phlegm. Nourishes and moistens the five *zang* organs. (*Koho-Yakugi*)

Used in Kampo prescriptions:
Sho-Kenchu-To, Dai-Kenchu-To.

地骨皮

MATRIMONY VINE

Solanaceae, *Lycium chinense* MILL.
Common name: Matrimony vine, Chinese Wolfberry
Japanese pronunciation: Jikoppi

Background: In the Orient this is a traditional tonic for the liver and kidneys; it nourishes semen, and improves vision. Also used for dizziness, headaches, lumbago, and diabetes.

KAMPO: The root bark of this plant is used today in Japan. (*Lycii Radix Cortex*)

Main constituents: Betaine, sitosterol, linolenic acid.

Used in Kampo prescriptions:
Jiin-Shiho-To, Seishin-Renshi-In.

黄　耆

MILK-VETCH

Leguminosae, *astragalus membranaceus* Bge.
Common name: Milk-vetch root
Japanese pronunciation: Ōgi

Background: Historically this root was used as a diuretic, to tone up the system, heal stubborn abcesses and facial swelling, and to heal diabetics. The drug is also cardiotonic, lowers blood pressure and blood sugar, and improves circulation in the skin.

KAMPO: The root is used. (*Astragali Radix*)

Main constituents: Flavonoids: formononetin, 3′-hydroxyformonoetin, 2′, 3-dihydroxy-7, 4′-dimethoxyisoflavone. Sugars: D-glucose, D-fructose, sucrose. Saponins: astragaloside I–VIII, soyasaponin I. Other: linoleic acid, linoleinic acid, β-sitosterol, choline, Y-aminobutyric acid.

Pharmacological properties: Hypotensive, peripheral blood vessel dilating, antiallergic, diuretic, tonic action, interferon inducing.

Usage according to Japanese classics: Used mainly to treat fluid in the skin (perspiration disorders, edema, etc.). Also used to treat yellow sweat (seen in cases where there is joint inflammation and general edema), night sweat, edema, and swelling if paralysis is present. (*Yakucho*)

Used in Kampo prescriptions:
Ogi-Kenchu-To, Kami-Kihi-To, Kihi-To, Shichimotsu-Koka-To, Juzen-Taiho-To, Seisho-Ekki-To, Seishin-Renshi-In, Dai-Bofu-To, Toki-To, Toki-Inshi, Ninjin-Yoei-To, Hange-Byakujutsu-Temma-To, Boi-Ogi-To, Hochu-Ekki-To.

荊　芥

MINT

Labiatae, *Schizonepeta tenuifolia* Briq. var. *japonica* Kitagawa.
Common name: Spring mint
Japanese pronunciation: Keigai

Background: The Romans crowned themselves with mint leaves and thought it the loveliest of herbs. The Greeks believed it could cure hiccups and counteract sea serpent stings. In much of the ancient world it was a symbol of hospitality. By the 18th century it had become a popular and important medicinal herb. The Japanese mint was thought to have antifertility properties. The menthol in mint gives it many other beneficial effects.

KAMPO: The flowering heads are used. (*Schizonepetae Spica*)

Main constituents: Essential oils: menthone, limonene, pulegone, Flavonoids: shizomepetoside A, B, C.

Pharmacological properties: Analgesic, anti-inflammatory, inhibits cyclic AMP.

Used in Kampo prescriptions:
Keigai-Rengyo-To, Jumi-Haidoku-To, Shofu-San, Sei-Jo-Bofu-To, Senkyu-Chacho-San, Ji-Zuso-Ippo, Toki-Inshi, Bofu-Tsusho-San.

薄荷

PEPPERMINT

Labiatae, *Mentha arvensis* L. var. *piperascens* MALINVAUD.
Common name: Peppermint
Japanese pronunciation: Hakka

Background: Peppermint has been used in the West for thousands of years for both medicinal and culinary purposes. Along with spearmint and cornmint, peppermint is used as a pain reliever, muscle relaxant, stimulant, tonic and carminative for various disorders: indigestion, nausea, diarrhea, sore throat, colds, headache, toothache, insomnia, cramps, liver ailments, heartburn and migraine among others. In Japan, peppermint's close relative—cornmint—is easier to obtain and also has germ-killing properties. Therefore, it can be substituted for peppermint.

KAMPO: The whole above-ground part of the plant is used. (*Menthae Herba*)

Main constituents: Essential oils: i-methol, acetylmenthol, i-menthone, α-pinene, camphene, i-limonene. Bitter constituents: piperitone, piperitenone, pulegone.

Pharmacological properties: Central nervous system suppressant, anticonvulsive dilates the peripheral blood vessels.

Usage according to Japanese classics: Used to treat light infectious diseases, and diseases caused by cold. It freshens the breath and can be used as a wash for poison ivy rash. (*Ippondo-Yakusen*)

Used in Kampo prescriptions:
Kami-Shoyo-San, Keigai-Rengyo-To, Saiko-Seikan-To, Jiin-Shiho-To, Seijo-Bofu-To, Senkyu-Chacho-San, Bofu-Tsusho-San.

防　己

MOONSEED

Menispermaceae, *Sinomenium acutum* REHD. et WILS.
Common name: Moonseed
Japanese pronunciation: Bōi

Background: Like the moon, this plant has a light and a dark side. On the bright side, it is an effective diuretic and laxative, useful in treating a wide variety of ailments including tuberculosis, rheumatism and arthritis. The plant contains berberine and related alkaloids used in the treatment of many chronic illnesses. The root extract once served as a substitute for sarsaparilla in soft drinks.

On the dark side, the berries are poisonous. Excessive doses bring on an increased pulse rate and violent vomiting and purging.

KAMPO: The root and stem of the plant are used. (*Sinomeni Caulis et Rhizoma*)

Main constituents: Alkaloids: sinomenine, disinomenine, ainactine, tuduranine, acutmine, acutmidine, magnoflorine, tetrandrine, isotetrandrine. Other: β-sitosterol, stigmasterol.

Pharmacological properties: Anti-inflammatory, anti-allergic, immunosuppressing, interferon inducing, analgesic.

Usage according to Japanese classics: Used mainly to treat irregularities of the fluid metabolism. (*Yakucho*)

Used in Kampo prescriptions:
Sokei-Kakketsu-To, Boi-Ogi-To,
Moku-Boi-To.

茵蔯蒿

CHINESE MOXA WEED

Compositae, *Artemisia capillaris* THUNB.
Common name: Capillaris, Chinese moxa weed
Japanese pronunciation: Inchinkō

Background: Used as an effective remedy for jaundice. The drug also promotes secretion of bile. Diuretic, antipyretic.

KAMPO: The flowering heads are used. (*Artemisiae Capillaris Spica*)

Main constituents: Essential oils: capillarin, capillin, capillene, capillone, etc. Chromones: capillarisin, capillartemisin A, B, etc. Cromines: esculetin 6, 7-dimethyl ether, etc. Flavonoids: cirsilineol, cirsimaritin, etc.

Pharmacological properties: Cholygogous, hepatoprotective, anti-inflammatory, antibacterial.

Usage according to Japanese classics: Mainly used to treat jaundice. (*Yakucho*)

Used in Kampo prescriptions:
Inchinko-To, Inchin-Gorei-San.

艾 葉

MUGWORT

Compositae, *Artemisia princeps* Pamp. or A. *montana* Pamp.
Common name: Mugwort, Ghost-plant
Japanese pronunciation: Gaiyō

Background: The mugwort is a tall, soft green feathery plant with a lovely fragrance and little whirling balls for flowers. In China, mugwort wards off evil spirits if hung during the time of the Dragon Festival (the 5th day of the 5th moon). The rest of the year, this herb is used in moxibustion, a proven healing technique that orginated in China. A moxa, or wad of this weed is burned on the surface of the skin at a specific acupuncture point to produce a burn scab. The heat, combined with the effect of acupuncture helps work the cure. Of course, this is a method of treatment requiring much training and can only be done by professionals. Mugwort, combined with agrimony and chamomile, is also used in herbal baths to relieve muscle aches and to prevent sunstroke.

KAMPO: The leaves and small stems are used. (*Artemisiae Follum*)

Main constituents: Essential oils: cineol, α-thujone. Fatty acids: capric acid, palmitic acid, stearic acid. Tannin: caffetannin. Other: vitamins, arachinic acid, amylase, invertase, catalase, peroxydase.

Pharmacological properties: Anti-coagulant, interferon inducing, complement activating.

Usage according to Japanese classics: Used for diarrhea, hematemesis (vomiting blood), irregular hemorrhaging of the urogenital organs in women, leukorrhea, and abdominal pain. Also used in moxibustion. (*Koho-Yakugi*)

Used in Kampo prescriptions:
Kyuki-Kyogai-To.

桑白皮

MULBERRY

Moraceae, *morus bombycuis* KOIDZ.
Common name: Mulberry
Japanese pronunciation: Sōhakubi

KAMPO: The cortices of the roots of this plant are used. (*Mori Cortex*)

Main constituents: Flavonoids: morusin, cyclomorusin, sanggenon A-E, kuwanone A, B, C. Triterpenoids: α-amyrin, β-amyrin. Other: β-sitosterol, fatty acids.

Pharmacological properties: Antitussive, anti-inflammatory, interferon inducing, hypotensive.

Usage according to Japanese classics: Used mainly to treat coughs. (*Ippondo-Yakusen*)

Used in Kampo prescriptions:
Goko-To, Seihai-To

MUSHROOMS

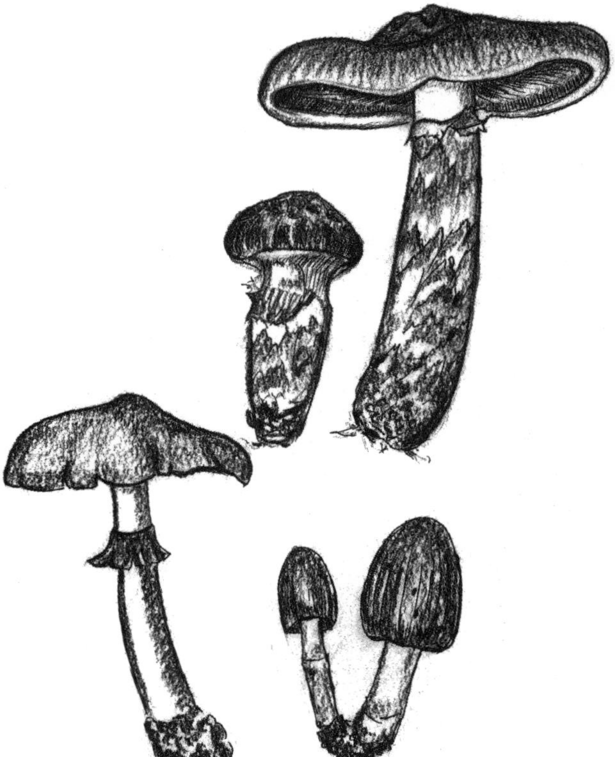

猪苓

UMBRELLA POLYPORE

Polyporaceae, *Polyporus umbellatus* FRIES.
Common name: Umbrella polypore
Japanese pronunciation: Chorei

Background: Gourmets acclaim mushrooms as a delicacy despite the fact they lack nutritive value except as a source of vitamin B. Mushrooms can be poisonous, especially the "destroying angel," *Amanita verna*. One Mexican mushroom contains psilocin and psilocylin which cause hallucinations. To make sure of getting the right mushroom for your kitchen—leave it to experts!

KAMPO: The whole mushroom is used in Kampo. (*Polyporus*)

Main constituents: Triterpenoids, sugars, ergosterol, 2-hydroxytertracosanic acid.

Pharmacological properties: Diuretic, reduces liver fat.

Usage according to Japanese classics: Used mainly to treat thirst and dysuria. (*Yakucho*)

Used in Kampo prescriptions:
Irei-To, Inchin-Gorei-San, Gorei-San,
Chorei-To, Chorei-To-Go-Shimotsu-To.

茯苓

FUNGI

Polyporaceae, *Poria cocos* WOLF.
Common name: Tuckahoe Indian Bread, Virginia Truffle, Orange Poria
Japanese pronunciation: Bukuryo

Background: This subterranean fungus has affinity for the heart, lungs, spleen, stomach and kidneys. It has been used traditionally as a diuretic, stomachic, and sedative.

KAMPO: This fungus is used with most of the skin removed. (*Hoelen*)

Main constituents: Sugars: pachyman. Terpenoids: eburicoic acid, pachymic acid, dehydroeburicoic acid, 3 β-o-acetyltumulosic acid, 3 β-o-acetyltdehydrotumulosic acid. Sterols: ergosterol.

Pharmacological properties: Diuretic, anti-gastric ulcer, hypoglycemic, anticoagulant, immunomoderating.

Usage according to Japanese classics: Used mainly to treat palpitations and muscle spasms. Also to treat dysuria, vertigo, discomfort, and restlessness. (*Yakucho*)

Used in Kampo prescriptions:
Irei-To, Inchin-Gorei-San, Kami-Kihi-To, Kami-Shoyo-San, Kihi-To, Keishi-Bukuryo-Gan, Keishi-Bukuryo-Gan-Ka-Yokuinin, Keihi-To, Gosha-Jinki-Gan, Goshaku-San, Gorin-San, Gorei-San, Saiko-Ka-Ryukotsu-Borei-To, Saiboku-To, Sairei-To, Sansonin-To, Jiin-Shiho-To, Shikunshi-To, Juzen-Taiho-To, Jumi-Haidoku-To, Sho-Hange-Ka-Bukuryo-To, Jinso-In, Shimbu-To, Seishin-Renshi-In, Seihai-To, Sokei-Kakketsu-To, Chikujo-Untan-To, Choto-San, Chorei-To, Chorei-To-Go-Shimotsu-To, Toki-Shakuyaku-San, Nijutsu-To, Nichin-To, Ninjin-Yoei-To, Hachimi-Jio-Gan, Hange-Koboku-To, Hange-Byakujutsu-Temma-To, Bukuryo-In, Bukuryo-In-Go-Hange-Koboku-To, Yoku-Kan-San, Yoku-Kan-San-Ka-Chimpi-Hange, Rikkunshi-To, Ryo-Kan-Kyo-Mi-Shin-Ge-Nin-To, Ryo-Kyo-Jutsu-Kan-To, Ryo-Kei-Jutsu-Kan-To, Rokumi-Gan.

川 芎

NETTLE

Umbelliferae, *Cnidium officinale* MAKINO.
Common name: Nettle
Japanese pronunciation: Senkyū
KAMPO: The rhizome of this plant is used. (*Cnidii Rhizoma*)

Main constitution: Cnidium. Essential oils: ligustilide, cnidilide, neocnidillide, butylphthalide, butylidenephthalid.

Pharmacolgical properties: Central nervous system suppressant, muscle relaxant, hypertensive (in small quantities), hypotensive (in large quantities), dilates the peripheral blood vessels, antithrombotic, antispasmodic, anti-tumor, increases skin temperature.

Usage according to Japanese classics: Used to treat various skin ailments caused by venereal disease: purulence, scabies, carbuncles, etc. Expels purulence and is good for eye diseases, headaches, weak legs and lower back, cramps in the extremities, purulence and blood in the urine; menstrual irregularities, retention of afterbirth, abdominal pain from difficult childbirth, labor pains, stagnant pathogens and pain in the muscles and bones. Breaks up stagnant blood and helps the circulation. (*Ippondo-Yakusen*)

Used in Kampo prescriptions:
Unkei-To, Unsei-In, Kakkon-To-Ka-Senkyu-Shin'i, Kyuki-Kyogai-To, Keigai-Rengyo-To, Goshaku-San, Saiko-Seikan-To, Sansonin-To, Shichimotsu-Koka-To, Shimotsu-To, Juzen-Taiho-To, Jumi-Haidoku-To, Sei-Jo-Bofu-To, Senkyu-Chacho-San, Sokei-Kakketsu-To, Dai-Bofu-To, Ji-Zuso-Ippo, Ji-Daboku-Ippo, Chorei-To-Go-Shimotsu-To, Toki-Inshi, Toki-Shakuyaku-San, Nyoshin-San, Bofu-Tsusho-San, Yoku-Kan-San, Yoku-Kan-San-Ka-Chimpi-Hange.

香附子

NUT-GRASS

Cyperaceae, *Cyperus rotundus* L.
Common name: Nut-grass
Japanese pronunciation: Kōbushi

Background: This is a common grass that grows on every continent except Africa. Commonly used by native herbalists.

KAMPO: The roots are used with rootlets removed. (*Cyperi Rhizoma*)

Main constitution: Seoqueterpene: cyperene, cyperol, isocyperol. Homoterpene: 1-α-pinene, cineol. Other: D-glucose, D-fructose, fatty oils.

Pharmacolgical properties: Inhibits the production of prostaglandin.

Usage according to Japanese classics: Used to treat chi'i stagnant in the epigastrium; discomfort and distention of the epigastrium. (*Ippondo-Yakusen*)

Used in Kampo prescriptions:
Koso-San, Goshaku-San, Jiin-Shiho-To, Senkyu-Chacho-San, Chikujo-Untan-To, Nijutsu-To, Nyoshin-San.

ORANGES

Everyone seems to love oranges, satsumas, and tangerines, but they don't love migraine sufferers. They are also among the few fruits contra-indicated in cases of arthritis. For the rest of us they are delicious. (Note: Grapefruits do not give us the same trouble.)

Orange-flower water was used in the past to treat "hysteria" because of its slightly relaxing effect. The leaves are anti-spasmodic and may be used to treat insomnia and epilepsy.

The bitter orange is the one used in marmalade. The dried peel of the sweet orange is used by Chinese herbalists as a diuretic and for its digestive properties.

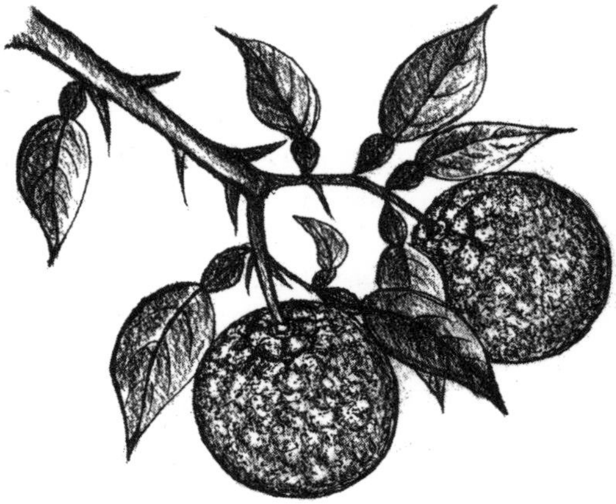

陳　皮

MANDARIN ORANGE

Rutaceae, *Citrus unshiu* MARKOV.
Common name: Mandarin Orange
Japanese pronunciation: Chinpi

KAMPO: The skin of the fruit is used. (*Aurantii Nobilis Pericarpium*)

Main constituents: Essential oils: α-limonine, auraptene, auraptin, linalool, terpineol. Favon-glycosides: hesperidin, naringin, nobiletin. Other: synephrine.

Pharmacological properties: Central nervous system suppressant, anti-inflammatory, anti-allergic, anti-convulsive.

Used in Kampo prescriptions:
Irei-To, Keihi-To, Koso-San, Goshaku-San, Jiin-Koka-To, Jiin-Shiho-To, Jinso-In, Shimpi-To, Seisho-Ekki-To, Seihai-To, Sokei-Kakketsu-To, Hange-Byakujutsu-Temma-To, Bukuryo-In, Bukuryo-In-Go-Hange-Koboku-To, Heii-San, Hochu-Ekki-To, Yoku-Kan-San-Ka-Chimpi-Hange, Rikkunshi-To.

枳　実

BITTER ORANGE

Rutaceae, *Citrus aurantium* L. var. *daidai* MAKINO, C. *natsudaidai* HAYATA, C. *unshiu* MARKOV.
Common name: Bitter orange
Japanese pronunciation: Kijitsu

KAMPO: The unripened fruit is used. (*Aurantii Fructus Immaturus*)

Main constituents: Essential oils: δ-limonene, linalcol, citral. Flavonoids: hesperidin, naringin. Cromines: umbelliferone, auraptene. Other: synephrine, citric acid.

Pharmacological properties: Muscle relaxant; anti-allergic.

Usage according to Japanese classics: Used mainly to treat pathogens that are stagnant within the body. Also to treat a feeling of distention and fullness in the chest; pain and a blocked feeling in the chest; pain and distention in the abdomen. (*Yakucho*)

Used in Kampo prescriptions:
Keigai-Rengyo-To, Goshaku-San, Shigyaku-San, Juncho-To, Jinso-In, Sei-Jo-Bofu-To, Dai-Saiko-To, Sai-Joki-To, Chikujo-Untan-To, Tsu-Do-San, Haino-San-Kyu-To, Bukuryo-In, Bukuryo-In-Go-Hange-Koboku-To, Mashinin-Gan.

桃仁

PEACH

Rosaceae, *Prunus persica* BATSCH or P. *persica* BATSCH var. *davidiana* MAXIM.
Common name: Peach
Japanese pronunciation: Tōnin

Background: Surprise! The common peach is effective against high blood pressure and chronic appendicitis. It also promotes circulation, dissolves clots, and acts as a laxative, emollient, and anti-tussive. High doses of the pit kernels are toxic according to the native herbal healers of China.

KAMPO: The seed is used. (*Persicae Semen*)

Main constituents: Fatty oils, hydrocyanic glyco side (amygdalin), emulsin, soluble proteins.

Pharmacological properties: Anticoagulant, antiallergic, anti-inflammatory, beneficial for climacteric disorders.

Usage according to Japanese classics: Used mainly to treat stagnant blood, and pain and distention in the lower abdomen. Also used to treat appendicitis and other inflammations of the organs in the lower abdomen, as well as menstrual irregularities. (*Yakucho*)

Used in Kampo prescriptions:
Keishi-Bukuryo-Gan, Keishi-Bukuryo-Gan-Ka-Yokuinin, Juncho-To, Sokei-Kakketsu-To, Daio-Botampi-To, Tokaku-Joki-To.

芍 薬

PEONY

Paeoniaceae, *Paeonia lactiflora* PALL.
Common name: Peony
Japanese pronunciation: Shakuyaku

Background: The peony ranks among the most beautiful of all plants. Herbal healers also insist that it is a wonderful tonic for the liver, blood, uterus and skin. Traditionally, it is used as a liver tonic and blood purifier, and as a cure for female complaints. It is also useful in treating anemia.

KAMPO: The root is used. (*Paeoniae Radix*)

Main constituents: Monoterpene glycosides: paeoniflorin, oxypaeoniflorin, benzoylpaeoniflorin, albiflorin. Other: paenol and its glycoside paeonoside, tannin, sucrose.

Pharmacological properties: Sedative, antispasmodic, analgesic, dilates the peripheral blood vessels, anti-inflammatory, anti-allergic, immunomoderating, promotes peristalsis, anti-gastric ulcer, antibacterial, BUN reducing.

Usage according to Japanese classics: Used mainly to treat stiff and cramped muscles; also to treat abdominal pain, headaches, numbness, pain, abdominal distention, coughing, diarrhea, and purulent swelling. (*Yakucho*)

Used in Kampo prescriptions:
Unkei-To, Ogi-Kenchu-To, Kakkon-To, Kakkon-To-Ka-Senkyu-Shin'i, Kami-Shoyo-San, Kyuki-Kyogai-To, Keigai-Rengyo-To, Keishi-To, Keishi-Ka-Shakuyaku-To, Keishi-Ka-Shakuyaku-Daio-To, Keishi-Ka-Jutsubu-To, Keishi-Ka-Ryukotsu-Borei-To, Keishi-Bukuryo-Gan, Keishi-Bukuryo-Gan-Ka-Yokuinin, Goshaku-San, Gorin-San, Saiko-Keishi-To, Saiko-Seikan-To, Jiin-Koka-To, Jiin-Shiho-To, Shigyaku-San, Shichimotsu-Koka-To, Shimotsu-To, Shakuyaku-Kanzo-To, Juzen-Taiho-To, Sho-Kenchu-To, Sho-Seiryu-To, Shoma-Kakkon-To, Shimbu-To, Sokei-Kakketsu-To, Dai-Saiko-To, Dai-Bofu-To, Chorei-To-Go-Shimotsu-To, Toki-Inshi, Toki-Kenchu-To, Toki-Shigyaku-Ka-Goshuyu-Shokyo-To, Toki-Shakuyaku-San, Toki-To, Ninjin-Yoei-To, Haino-San-Kyu-To, Bofu-Tsusho-San, Mashinin-Gan, Yokuinin-To.

牡丹皮

GIANT PEONY

Paeoniaceae, *Paeonis suffruticosa* ANDR.
Common name: Giant peony
Japanese pronunciation: Botanpi

KAMPO: The skin of the root is used. (*Moutan Cortex*)

Main constituents: Monoterpene glycosides: paeoniflorin, oxypaeoniflorin, benzoylpaeoniflorin. Phenols: paenol, oxypaeoniflorin, benzoylpaeoniflorin. Phenols: paenol, paeonoside, paeonolids. Other: tannins (δ-catechin), sucrose.

Pharmacological properties: Analgesic, sedative, anti-inflammatory, anti-allergic, immunomoderating, fat-metabolism suppressant, anticoagulant, antibacterial, antiviral, improves dismenorrhea.

Usage according to Japanese classics: Used in cases of hardened, stagnant blood and purulent swelling. Aids menstrual flow, reduces bruises and sprains. Relieves lower back pain and severe, restless fever. (*Koho-Yakugi*)

Used in Kampo prescriptions:
Unkei-To, Keishi-Bukuryo-Gan, Keishi-Bukuryo-Gan-Ka-Yokuinin, Goshaku-Jinki-Gan, Daio-Botampi-To, Hachimi-Jio-Gan, Rokumi-Gan.

半 夏

PINELLIA

Araceae, *Pinellia ternata* BREIT.
Common name: Pinellia
Japanese pronunciation: Hange

Background: This herb is considered, traditionally, to have an affinity for the spleen and stomach. It has been used for thousands of years as an expectorant and anti-emetic. Caution: Pregnant women should use herb sparingly; the fresh herb is slightly toxic, but the dried is not. The toxin is neutralized with tea.

KAMPO: The tuber is used. (*Pipelliae Tuber*)

Main constituents: Phenyls: homogentistic cid, 3,4-hydroxybenzaldehyde. Alkaloids: *l*-ephedrine. Amino acids: arginine, aspartic acid. Other: starch, essential oils, β-sitosterol, palmitic acid.

Pharmacological properties: Central nervous system suppressant, analgesic, anti-emetic, antispasmodic, anti-peptic ulcer, increases mucus secretion, stimulates peristalsis, immunomoderating.

Usage according to Japanese classics: Used mainly to treat stagnant fluids, irregularities of the fluid metabolism, and vomiting. Also used to treat chest pain, distention of the chest and abdomen, sore throat, cough, palpitations, and borborygm. (*Yakucho*)

Used in Kampo prescriptions:
Unkei-To, Oren-To, Goshaku-San, Saikan-To, Saiboku-To, Sairei-To, Saiko-Ka-Ryukotsu-Borei-To, Saiko-Keishi-To, Sho-Saiko-To, Sho-Saiko-To-Ka-Kikyo-Sekko, Sho-Seiryu-To, Sho-Hange-Bukuryo-To, Jinso-In, Dai-Saiko-To, Chikujo-Untan-To, Choto-San, Toki-To, Nijutsu-To, Nichin-To, Bakumondo-To, Hange-Koboku-To, Hange-Shashin-To, Yoku-Kan-San-Ka-Chimpi-Hange, Rikkunshi-To, Ryo-Kan-Kyo-Mi-Shin-Ge-Nin-To.

車前子

PLANTAIN

Plantaginaceae, *Plantago asiatica* L.
Common name: Plantago, Plantain
Japanese pronunciation: Shazenshi

Background: Plantain has been called the "mother of herbs." In Old World traditional medicine it was used as a remedy for cuts, sores, burns, snake bites, insect bites, and inflammations. A tea brewed from the leaves was also common remedy for diarrhea, dysentery, and bleeding from mucous membranes. The Chinese tell us that it is the only diuretic that also tonifies the kidneys. They also use it in many aphrodisiac prescriptions. The seeds—known as psyllium seeds in the U.S.—are a useful bulk laxative, one half ounce taken with a cup of hot water.

KAMPO: The seed is used. (*Plantaginis Semen*)

Main constituents: Plantasan aucubin, disaccharide, fatty acids.

Pharmacological properties: Interferon inducing.

Usage according to Japanese classics: Used to help the function of the urinary tract. Relieves dysuria and urinary irregularities in pregnant women. Helps to lubricate during childbirth and relieves swelling. (*Ippondo-Yakusen*)

Used in Kampo prescriptions:
Gosha-Jinki-Gan, Gorin-San, Seishin-Renshi-In, Ryutan-Shakan-To.

大　黄

RHUBARB

Polygonaceae, *Rhem palmatum* L., R. *tanguticum* MAXIM, R. *officinale* BAILL.
Common name: Turkey rhubarb, Chinese rhubarb
Japanese pronunciation: Daiō

Background: This herbal, native to the mountainious areas of western China and Tibet, has been used medicinally for more than 2,000 years. Yet its components seem diametrically opposed! Its anthraglycosides have laxative effects; its tannins are astringents. Hence, depending upon the size of the dose and the way it is given, the rhizome is effective in treating both constipation and diarrhea. In Kampo it is used primarily as a laxative.

KAMPO: The root is used. (*Rhei Rhizoma*)

Main constituents: Anthraquinenes: emodin, rhein, aloe-emodin, chrysophanol, physcion. Dianthrones: sennoside A-F, sennidin A. Phenol glycosides: lindleyin Tannins: rhatannin. Other: gallic acid, cinnamic acid.

Pharmacological properties: Laxative, antibacterial, reduces BUN, anticoagulant, anti-inflammatory, antimutagenic, interferon inducing.

Usage according to Japanese classics: Used mainly to purge (as a laxative) pathogens from the body. Relieves distention of the chest and abdomen, abdominal pain, constipation and dysuria. Also used to treat jaundice and stagnant blood. (*Yakucho*)

Used in Kampo prescriptions:
Inchinko-To, Otsuji-To, Keishi-Ka-Shakuyaku-Daio-To, San'o-Shashin-To, Juñcho-To, Daio-Kanzo-To, Daio-Botampi-To, Dai-Saiko-To, Dai-Joki-To, Ji-Daboku-Ippo, Ji-Zuso-Ippo, Choi-Joki-To, Tsu-Do-San, Tokaku-Joki-To, Bofu-Tsusho-San, Mashinin-Gan.

粳 米

RICE

Gramineae, *Oryza sativa* L.
Common name: Brown rice
Japanese pronunciation: Kōbei (Genmai)

Background: In China, India, and Japan the word for rice is synonymous with the word for "food." It is considered to be the specific grain for strengthening the lungs. Hearty brown rice strengthens the body and constitution and is the basic food of people living throughout the Far East, including our own Zen temples here in Japan. Brown rice is recommended especially during the winter month because it is a warming food.

KAMPO: The whole grain of this plant is used with the hull removed. (*Oryza sativa*)

Main constituents: Starch, dextrin.

Pharmacological properties: Prevents the loss of body fluids and stops thirst, if used regularly in the diet it keeps the body healthy. (*Ippondo-Yakusen*)

Used in Kampo prescriptions:
Bakumondo-To, Byakko-Ka-Ninjin-To.

五味子

SCHISANDRA

Schisandraceae, *Schisandra chinensis* BAILL.
Common name: Schisandra
Japanese pronunciation: Gomishi

KAMPO: The fruit is used. (*Schisandrae Fructus*)

Main constituents: Essential oils: citral, β-chamigren, β-chamigrenal, sesquicarene. Lignin derivatives: schizanfrin A-D, deoxyschizandrin, gomisin A-D, F-H, J, pregomisin. Organic acids: citric acid, malic acid, tartaric acid, protocatechuic acid, ascorbic acid.

Pharmacological properties: Sedative, anti-convulsive, anti-tussive, analgesic, anti-gastric ulcer, hepatoprotective.

Usage according to Japanese classics: Used mainly to treat coughing and hood-vertigo (a feeling of constriction like a band around the head, accompanied by a heavy feeling in the head). (*Yakucho*)

Used in Kampo prescription:
Sho-Seiryu-To, Seisho-ekki-To, Sei-Hai-To, Ninjin-Yoei-To, Ryo-Kan-Kyo-Mi-Shin-Ge-Nin-To.

黄芩

SKULLCAP

Labiatae, *Scutellaria baicalensis* GEORGI.
Common name: Baical skullcap root/scute.
Japanese pronunciation: Ōgon

Background: Skullcap, which acts as a tonic, a sedative, and an anti-spasmodic, helps to strengthen and support the nervous system. Skullcap has been used to treat a wide range of nervous disorders including migraine, depression, anxiety, insomnia, and neuralgia. In ancient times, skullcap was also used for treating epilepsy and rabies. Care should be taken with this drug as large doses can cause dizziness, erratic pulse rate, and mental confusion. Its bitter taste is also strengthening and stimulating to the digestion.

KAMPO: The root is used with the skin removed. (*Scutellariae Radix*)

Main constituents: Flavonoids: baicalin, baicalein, wogonin, wogonin glucuronids, oroxylin A, skullcapflavone. Steroids: β-sitosterol, campesterol. Sugars: sucrose, D-glucose.

Pharmacological properties: Cholagogous, laxative, hepatoprotective, anti-tussive toxic, diuretic, anti-inflammatory, anti-allergic, anti-arteriosclerosis, hypotensive, anti-spasmodic, prevents the production of prostaglandin.

Usage according to Japanese classics: Used mainly to treat discomfort in the epigastrium. Also used to treat distention of the hypochondrium, vomiting and diarrhea. (*Yakucho*)

Used in Kampo prescriptions:
Unsei-In, Otsuji-To, Oren-Gedoku-To, Keigai-Rengyo-To, Gorin-San, Saikan-To, Saiko-Ka-Ryukotsu-Borei-To, Saiko-Keishi-To, Saiko-Seikan-To, Saiboku-To, Sairei-To, San'o-Shashin-To, Sammotsu-Ogon-To, Sho-Saiko-To, Sho-Saiko-To-Ka-Kiyo-Sekko, Juncho-To, Shin'i-Seihai-To, Sei-Jo-Bofu-To, Seishin-Renshi-In, Seihai-To, Dai-Saiko-To, Nijutsu-To, Nyoshin-San, Hange-Shashin-To, Bofu-Tsusho-San, Ryutan-Shakan-To.

栝楼根

SNAKE GOURD

Curcurbitaceae, *Trichosanthes kirillowii* MAXIM. var. *japonicum* KITAM., T. *bracteata* VOIGT or T. *kirillowii* MAXIM.
Common name: Snake gourd root
Japanese pronunciation: Karokon

Background: The root of this plant is antipyretic and promotes lactation. It has an affinity for the lungs, stomach, and large intestine.

KAMPO: The peeled root of this plant is used. (*Trichosanthis Radix*)

Main constituents: Starch, trichosanic acid, amino acids.

Pharmacological properties: Anti-peptic ulcer, interferon inducing.

Usage according to Japanese classics: Used mainly to treat thirst. (*Yakucho-Zokuhen*)

Used in Kampo prescriptions:
Saiko-Keishi-Kankyo-To, Saiko-Seikan-To.

沢 瀉

WATER PLANTAIN

Alismataceae, *Alisma orientale* JUZPEC.
Common name: Water Plantain
Japanese pronunciation: Takusha

Background: Traditionally used in the Orient for problems of the kidneys and bladder. Also has a strong affinity for the female genitalia.

KAMPO: The rhizome of this plant is used. (*Alismatis Rhizoma*)

Main constituents: Alistol A, B, C and acetate. Sugars: D-glucose, D-fructose, sucrose. Other: β-sitosterol, amino acids, lecithin, choline, K salt, vitamins, starch.

Pharmacological properties: Diuretic, anti-fatty liver, reduces the amount of cholesterol in the blood, anticoagulant.

Usage according to Japanese classics: Used mainly to treat dysuria and hood vertigo. Also relieves thirst. (*Yakucho*)

Used in Kampo prescriptions:
Irei-To, Inchin-Gorei-San, Keihi-To, Gosha-Jinki-Gan, Gorin-San, Gorei-San, Sairei-To, Toki-Shakuyaku-San, Chorei-To, Ryutan-Shakan-To. Rokumi-Gan.

冬瓜子

WINTER MELON

Curcurbitaceae, *Benincasa cerifera* SAVI or B. *cerifera* SAVI forms *emarginata* K. KIMURA et S. SUGIYAMA.
Common name: Winter Melon, Wax Gourd (Muskmelon)

KAMPO: The seeds are used. (*Benincasae Semen*)

Main constituents: Fatty oils: oleic acid, linoleic acid. Other: adenine, trigonelline.

Pharmacological properties: Immunomoderating, anti-tumor.

Usage according to Japanese classics: Used mainly to treat edema due to irregularities of the circulatory system. (*Ippondo-Yakusen*)

Used in Kampo prescriptions:
Daio-Botampi-To.

山 薬

YAM

Dioscoreaceae, Dioscorea japonica THUMB, or *Dioscorea batatas* DECNE.
Common name: Yam
Japanese pronunciation: Sanyaku

Background: One of the great breakthroughs of medical science was made in the '30s when scientists began searching for cortisone and sex hormones in nature. Eventually, yams were found to be an excellent source of diosgenin, the basic substance from which birth control pills and several other steroid drugs are made.

KAMPO: The rhizome of this plant is used with the skin removed. (*Dioscoreae Rhizoma*)

Main constituents: Sugars, starch, protein. Other: amino acids, choline, allantoin.

Pharmacological properties: Increases the production of male hormones.

Usage according to Japanese classics: Used to stop diarrhea. (*Ippondo-Yakusen*)

Used in Kampo prescriptions:
Keihi-To, Gosha-Jinki-Gan, Hachimi-Jio-Gan, Rokumi-Gan.

DRAGON BONES

Thousands of years ago Chinese "barefoot doctors" had to pass along their knowledge without written records. This, of course, led to a great deal of superstition and symbolism being added to herbalism by villagers. When Chinese herbal medicine reached Japan, it was still riddled with animal and mineral drugs, and combinations of them selected for their emblematic significance rather than medicinal properties. All of this lore and symbolism has been severely questioned in modern times with some surprising results. Although many apparently quack remedies have been eliminated, many also are proving their value in the best, most modern laboratories. In 1983, for example, a 400-year-old prescription for the treatment of hemorrhoids was tested on 40,000 patients in Beijing and was proven to be 90% effective. The remedy? An injection of insect secretions on sumac leaves mixed with crystal salt!

That is why our Kampo doctors still may turn to fossil bones and oyster shells for cures, or to verdigris, bear's gall, and turtle shell, donkey's skin, or to minerals. Even if you credit the cure to their value as a placebo, should we not be grateful that they do effect a cure? Without apology then, we list a few of the more exotic items in our shelves. I treasure them, because they always remind me how far we have gone in herbal medicine since those early days.

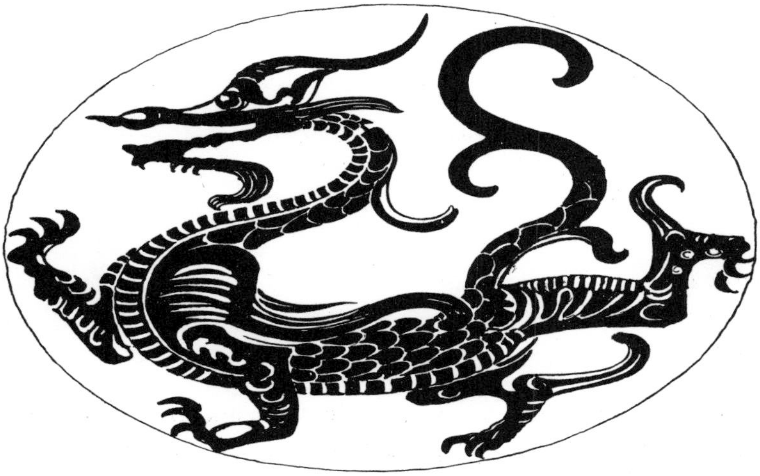

竜 骨

FOSSIL BONES

Fossilia Ossis Mastodi
Common name: Dragon bones, Fossil bones
Japanese pronunciation: Ryūkotsu

Background: Evidence does indicate that this remedy works in cases of hypertension, insomnia, shock, fright, hysteria, dizziness, spermatorrhea, leukorrhea, and diarrhea. Also has effective external styptic action on abcesses and other persistent sores.

KAMPO: The fossilized bones of large animals are used for their content of calcium carbonate.

Main constituents: calcium carbonate, calcium phosphate, and other inorganic substances, organic acids, amino acids.

Usage according to Japanese classics: Used mainly in cases of palpitations below the umbilicus. Also for nervousness, spermatorrhea, and nocturnal emission. (*Yakucho*)

Used in Kampo prescriptions:
Keishi-Ka-Ryukotsu-Borei-To, Saiko-Ka-Ryukotsu-Borei-To.

熊 胆

BEAR GALL

Ursidae, *Ursus arctos* L.
Common name: Bear Gall
Japanese pronunciation: Yūtan

Main constituents: Biles: ursodeoxycholic acid, chenodeoxycholic acid, cholic acid, deoxycholic acid and their oxygen attached to taurine, etc.

Pharmacological properties: Cholygogous, dissolves gall stones, antispasmodic.

Usage according to Japanese classics: The dried content of gall bladder—*Fel Ursi*—is used to treat abdominal tumor, abdominal pain due to obstruction or bad food intake; cramps in neck and back; chest pains; unsuccessful urge to vomit; irritability; insanity; intermittent fever (malaria-like state); diarrhea. Kills parasitic insects, stops vomiting, diffuses smallpox. Also used to treat children's nervous breakdowns, convulsions, stomach ache during pregnancy, abdominal pain after childbirth, produce labor pains. Clears blurred eyes, stops pain of hemorrhoids. Restores vitality, and rids impurities from body. (*Ippondo-Yakusen*)

蟬 退

CICADA

Cicadidae, *Cryptotympana* pustulata FABR.
Common name: Cicada
Japanese pronunciation: Zentai

KAMPO: The cast-off shell or the skin of the cicada is used. (*Cicadae periostracus*)

Main constituents: Chitin, etc.

Pharmacological properties: Interferon inducing.

Used in Kampo prescriptions:
Shofu-San.

䗪 虫

EUPOLYPHAGA

Blattidae, *Eupolyphaga sinensis* WALKER, *Opisthoplatia orientalis* BURM.
Common name: Eupolyphaga
Japanese pronunciation: Shachu

KAMPO: The whole body of the female insect is used. (*Eupolyphaga*)

Pharmacological properties: Anti-coagulant, hepatoprotective.

Usage according to Japanese classics: Used mainly to dissolve blood clots, and improve stagnant circulation. Also to treat pain due to heaviness in the abdomen and irregular menstrual cycle. (*Yakusen-Zokuhen*)

小 麦

WHEAT

Gramineae, *Triticum sativum* Lam.
Common name: Wheat
Japanese pronunciation: Shōbaku

KAMPO: The seeds of this plant are used. (*Tritici Fructus*)

Main constituents: Sugars, arginine, dextrin, fats, proteins, etc.

Usage according to Japanese classics: Used to remove discomforting stuffiness. Stops thirst and dryness of the mouth. Improves urine discharge and stimulates mental activities. (*Koho-Yakugi*)

Used in Kampo prescriptions:
Kam-Baku-Taiso-To.

牡 蛎

OYSTER

Osteridae, *Ostrea gigas* Thunb.
Common name: Oyster shell
Japanese pronunciation: Borei

Background: The shell of the oyster contains a full 75% calcium carbonate; promotes bone growth; and overcomes calcium-deficiency in pregnant women. The shell also is used as a sedative, astringent, and to treat tumors, heart palpitations, insomnia, blurry vision, and a variety of other ills.

KAMPO: The shell is used. (*Ostreae Testa*)

Main constituents: $CaCo_3$, $Ca_3(PO_4)_2$ and the inorganic salts, amino acids, glycogen, betaine, taurin, and vitamins.

Usage according to Japanese classics: Used mainly to treat palpitations in the chest and abdomen. Also to treat mental anxiety and nervousness. (*Yakucho*)

Used in Kampo prescriptions:
Anchu-San, Keishi-Ka-Ryukotsu-Borei-To, Saiko-Keishi-Kankyo-To, Saiko-Ka-Ryukotsu-Borei-To.

阿 膠

DONKEY HIDE

Zoological name: Equidae, *Equus aninus* L.
Common name: Donkey hide
Japanese pronunciation: Akyō

Background: A gelatin is made from the skin of the donkey (Other parts of the animal and other animals may be used.)

Believe it or not, this has been used in the past for blood deficiency, sallow complexion, dizziness, heart palpitations, blood in stool, and insomnia.

KAMPO: The same gelatin is still used today in Kampo. (*Asini Gelatinum*)

Main constitutions: Collagen, glutin, chondrin, amino acids.

Pharmacological properties: It is known to have an anticoagulant effect.

Usage according to Japanese classics: Used mainly to treat various blood conditions (hemorrhaging, hematemesis, blood in the stool, irregular menstruation, blood stagnation, etc.). Also used for chest pains and insomnia. (*Yakubi-Zokuhen*)

Used in Kampo prescriptions:
Unkei-To, Kyuki-Kyogai-To, Sha-Kanzo-To, Chorei-To, Chorei-To-Go-Shimotsu-To.

滑　石

MINERALS

Talc (Hydrous Magnesium Silicate)
Japanese pronunciation: Kasseki

Background: Used as a diuretic, antiphlogistic, and refrigerant. Effective remedy for boils and prickly heat.

Usage according to Japanese classics: Used to treat scanty urine and difficulty in passing urine. Also used to treat thirst. (*Yakucho*)

Used in Kampo prescriptions:
Gorin-San, Chorei-To, Chorei-To-Go-Shimotsu-To, Bofu-Tsusho-San.

Mirabilite (Natrium Sulfuricum)
Japanese pronunciation: Bosho

Pharmacological properties: Laxative, anticoagulant.

Usage according to Japanese classics: Used mainly to soften hardness. Used to treat hardness of the epigastrium, severe pain upon pressure in the lower left abdomen, pain and distention of the epigastrium, dry hard stools, stagnant food in the digestive tract, abdominal distention, discomfort and tension of the lower abdomen, and other illnesses caused by stagnant pathogens. (*Yakucho*)

Used in Kampo prescriptions:
Daio-Botampi-To, Dai-Joki-To, Choi-Joki-To, Tsu-Do-San, Tokaku-Joki-To, Bofu-Tsusho-San.

Gypsum (Gypsum Fibrosum) $CaSO_4 \cdot 2H_2O$
Japanese pronunciation: Sekkō

Pharmacological properties: Stops thirst, diuretic.

Usage according to Japanese classics: Used mainly to treat severe thirst. Also used to treat delirium, distress, and general fever (covering the entire body). (*Yakucho*)

Used in Kampo prescriptions:
Eppi-Ka-Jutsu-To, Goko-To, Sho-Saiko-To-Ka-Kikyo-Sekko, Shofu-San, Shin'i-Seihai-To, Choto-San, Byakko-Ka-Ninjin-To, Bofu-Tsusho-San, Ma-Kyo-Kan-Seki-To.

Common Name Botanical Name Japanese Pronunciation	Pharmaceutical Name and Constituents	Pharmacological properties	Usage according to Japanese classics	Kampo prescriptions used in
APARAGUS Asparagus cochinchinensis MERR. Tenmondō	Asparagi Radix Saponin: Asp- IV, V, VI, VII Others: β-sitosterol starches. sugars. asparagine	Interferon inducing		JIIN-KOKA-TO, SEIHAI-TO
BALLOON FLOWER Platycodon grandiflorum A. DC. Kinkyō	Platycodi Radix Saponin: platycodin A, C, D, D_2, polygalacin D, D_2. Sterols: α-spinasterol. Triterpene: betulin. Other: inulin, platycodonin, vitamin A, arginine.	Analgesic, sedative, anti-pyretic, antitussive, anti-spasmodic, dilates the peripheral blood vessels, hypoglycemic, anti-ulcer, inhibits cyclic AMP.	Used mainly to treat sputum containing pus also boils, tumors and throat pains. (Yakucho)	KIKYO-TO, KEIGAI-RENGYO-TO, GOSHAKU-SAN, SAIKO-SEIKAN-TO, SHO-SAIKO-TO-KA-KIKYO-SEKKO, JUMI-HAIDOKU-TO, JINSO-IN, SEI-JO-BOFUTO, SEIHAI-TO, CHIKUJO-UNTAN-TO, HAINO-SAN-KYU-TO, BOFU-TSUSHO-SAN.
CALTROP Tribulus terrestris L. Shitsurishi	Tribuli Fructus Alkaloids: harmine, harmane Flavonoids: kampferol, astragalin, tribuloside. Other: tannin, essential oils	Antispasmodic		TOKI-INSHI.
CHINESE CORNBIND (Ho-shou-wu) Polygonom multiflorum THUNB. Kashū	Polygoni Multiflori Radix Anthraquinenes: emodin, physcion, chrysophanol. Other: stilbene glycoside.	Anti-hyperlipemia, hepatoprotective.		TOKI-INSHI.
CHINESE WOLFBERRY BOXTHORN Lycium chinense MILL. Kukoshi	Lucii Fructus Carotinoids: zeaxanthin, physalien. Other: betaine, β-sitosterol, linoleic acid.	Reduces cholesterol.		

EUCOMMIA Eucommia ulmoides OLIV. Tochū	Eucommiae Cortex Gutta-percha, pinoresinol-diglucoside, geniposice, geniposidic acid, ulmoprenol.	Hypotensive, anti-stress.		DAI-BOFU-TO
FRITILLARIA Fritillaria verticillata WILLD. var. thunbergii BAK. Temma	Fritillariae Bulbus Alkaloids: verticine, verticilline, fritillarine, peimine. Glucose: peiminoside (peimine plus D-glucose).	Hypotensive.	Used to treat colds in the chest and diaphram, stagnant fluids, and disorders due to stagnant fluids. (Yakucho)	JIIN-SHIHO-TO, SEIHAI-TO.
GASTROIA Gastrodia elata BL. Temma	Gastrodiae Tuber Essential oils: vanillin, vanillyl, alcohol. Others: vitamins.	Interferon inducing.		HANGE-BYAKUJUTSU-TEMMA-TO.
GLEHNIA Glehnia littoralis FR. SCHM-ex MIQ. Hamabōfū	Glehniae Radix cum Rhizoma Essential oils, croumarins, bitter constitution		Used to treat pain in joints due to colds: stagnant blood: headaches and dizziness; cramp pains in hands and feet. (Koho-Yakugi)	SEI-JO-BOFU-TO.
GREAT BURDOCK Arctium lappa L. Gobōshi	Arctii Fructus Lignin derivatives: artigenin, arctiin, lappaol A ~ E.	Contracts myoma of the uterus.	Used to treat obstruction in the throat, swellings, boils, tumors, and to relieve pain. (Ippondo-Yakusen)	SAIKO-SEIKAN-TO, SHOFU-SAN.
JAPANESE HONEYSUCKLE Lonicera japonica THUNB. Nindō	Lonicerae Caulis et Folium Tannin, bitter glucose, (loganin).	Improves fat metabolism.	Used to treat urine discharge. Also boils, tumors, abscess, and infected skin due to syphillis and gonorrhea, and infected urethra. (Ippondo-Yakusen)	JI-ZUSO-IPPO.

Common Name Botanical Name Japanese Pronunciation	Pharmaceutical Name and Constituents	Pharmacological properties	Usage according to Japanese classics	Kampo prescriptions used in
HOUTTUYNIA Houttuynia cordata THUNB. Jūyaku	Houttuyniae Herba Esential oils: decanolacetalehyde, methylknonylketone, α-pinene, limonene, Flavonoids: quercetin, quercitrin. Other: K-salt.	Central nervous system suppressant. Diuretic.		
LILY Lilium lancifolium THUNB, L. brownii F.E. BROWN var. cholchesteri WILS. Byakugō	Lilii Bulbus Starches, proteins, fats, alkaloids.			SHIN'I-SEIHAI-TO.
LITHOSPERMUM Lithospermum erythrorhizon SIEB. et ZUCC., Macrotomia euchroma PAULS. Shikon	Lithospermi Radix Pigments: shikonin, acetylshikonin, β-dimethylacrylshikonin. Hydrocyanic glycocides: lithospermoside. Other: lithospermic acid, allantoin, sugars.	Anti-inflammatory, inhibits the production of prostaglandin, antibacterial, anti-tumor, compliment activating, interferon inducing.		SHIUN-KO.
LONGAN Euphoria longana LAM. Ryugan'niku	Longanae Arillus Sugars, and organic acids such as tartaric acids.			KAMI-KIHI-TO, KIHI-TO.
LOQUAT Eriobotrya japonica LINDL. Biwayō	Eriobotryae Folium Triterpenoids: ursolic acid, oleanoli acid, 2 α-hydroxyoleanolic-acid-methyl-ester. Others: amygdalin, sugars, tannin, organic acids	Anti-inflammatory.	Used to treat vomiting, coughing. (Ippondo-Yakusen)	SHIN'I-SEIHAI-TO.

NUPHAR Nuphar japonicum DC.	Nupharis Rhizoma Alkaloids: nupharidine, deoxynupharidine, nupharamine. Other: β-sitosterol, oleic acid, palmitic acid, ellagic acid, nicotinic acid, tannin (nupharin A, B, C).	Tranquilizer: prevents the production of prostaglandin.	Used to resolve blood stagnation. Improves circulation. Also used to treat bruises, syphilis, and diseases due to stagnant blood after childbirth. (Ippondo-Yakusen)	JI-DABOKU-IPPO.
OAK BARK Quercus acutissima CARRUTH. Bokusō	Quercus Cortex Tannin, flavonoids (quercitrin). starches, sucrose, fats.		Used to treat blood stagnation, circulation disorders, venereal diseases, infected skin with pus discharge, and bruises. (Ippondo-Yakusen)	JUNI-HAIDOKU-TO, JI-DABOKU-IPPO.
PEUCEDANUM Peucedanum praeruptorum DUNN. Zenko	Peucedani Radix Croumarin (Pd- Ia, II, III, Ib, etc.) Croumarin derivatives: praeruptorin, decurside I ~ V, nodakenin, mannitol.	Anti-inflammatory, anti-tumor.	Used for fever and chills of infectious disease. Phlegm, obstruction in chest, boils, tumors, and vomiting and headaches. Resolves maldistribution of body fluids and improves stomach activity and food digestion. (Koho-Yakugi)	JINSO-IN.
PEUCEDANUM Peucedanum praeruptorum DUNN. Zenko	Polygalae Radix Saponin: Onjisaponin A-G. Other: Gentiopicroside, sugars, fatty oils.	Anti-peptic ulcer, anti-spasmodic, antimutagenic, interferon inducing.		KAMI-KIHI-TO, KIHI-TO, NINJIN-YOEI-TO
PURGING CROTON Croton tiglium L. Hazu	Crotonis Semen Croton oil: oleic acid, palmitic acid, stearic acid, lauric acid, crotonic acid. Others: phorbol ester, arginine.	Most poisonous of all strong purgatives. (Use with care.)	Used to treat constipation, cleanse intestines, and for stomach ache. Taboo for pregnant women. (Ippondo-Yakusen)	

Common Name Botanical Name Japanese Pronunciation	Pharmaceutical Name and Constituents	Pharmacological properties	Usage according to Japanese classics	Kampo prescriptions used in
SAFFLOWER Carthamus tinctorius L. Kōka	Carthami Flos Pigments: carthamin, saflor yellow. Flavonoids: carthamidin, neo carthamin. Other: essential oils, lignin.	Hypotensive, immunomoderating, anti-inflammatory.	Used to treat blood stasis and pain from clots. (Ippondo-Yakusen)	JI-ZUSO-IPPO, TSU-DO-SAN.
SAPPAN WOOD Caesalpinia sappan L. Soboku	Sappan Lignum Pigment (brasilin), tannin, berazilin.	Improves hyperlipopenia.		TSU-DO-SAN.
SESAME SEEDS Sesamum indicum L. Goma	Sesame Semen Fatty acids: linoleic acid, palmitic acid, steraic acid, oleic acid. Other: sesamin, semamol.			SHOFU—SAN, SHIUM—KO (Ointment containing sesame oil for external application.)
SNAKE GOURD Trichosanthes kirillowii MAXIM. var. T. bracteata VOIGT, T. kirillowii MAXIM. Karonin	Trichosanthis Semen Fatty oils: oleic acid, linolic acid, linolenic acid, trichosanic acid.	Immunomoderating.		SAIKAN-TO.
SOPHORA Sophora flavescens AIT. Kujin	Sophorae Radix Alkaloids: matrine, oxymatrine, sophoranol. Flavonoids: xanthohumol, kurarinone, kuraridin, kuraridinol, kurarinol.	Hypotensive, anti-peptic ulcer, hepatoprotective, interferon inducing.		SAMMOTSU-OGON-TO, SHOFU-SAN.
SPIKENARD (Rhizome/Root) Aralia cordata THUNB. Dokkatsu	Araliae Rhizoma et Radiz Essential oils, triterpenoids.	Used to treat pain and stiffness of muscles and joints, eye diseases, pain from swollen eyes, blurred vision, numbness, pruritus cutanea.		JUMI-HAIDOKU-TO.

SPIKENARD (Root)	Arliae Radix	Used when there is chill, numbness and pain caused by wind, cold or dampness. Relieves siffness in joints and muscles; eye problems: itchy skin and spasms. (Ippondo-Yakusen)		NIJUTSU-TO.
SWERTIA Swertia japonica MAKINO. Tōyaku	Swertiae Herba Bitter constituents: swertiamarin, sweroside, amaroside, gentiopieroside. Xanthorne derivatives: swertianin, norswertianin, swertianolin, bellidifolin. Others: olenolic acid, gentianin.	Increase secretion of digestive fluids.		
TEA Thea sinensis L. Chayo	Theae Folium Alkaloids: caffine, theophylline, xathine; Flavonoids: kaemphetrin, querctrtin. Essential oils: β-hexenal, isobutylaldehyde, butylic acid. Other: saponin, steroids, triterpenoids, amino acids, vitamins.	Central nervous system stimulant, prevents the breakdown of fats, obstruction of mutation.		SENKYU-CHACHO-SAN.
WILD TURNIP. Arisaema japonicum BL., A. Heterophyllum BR. Tennanshō	Arisaematis Tuber Saponin, starches, amino acids.			NIJUTSU-TO

PART FIVE

Kampo Medications

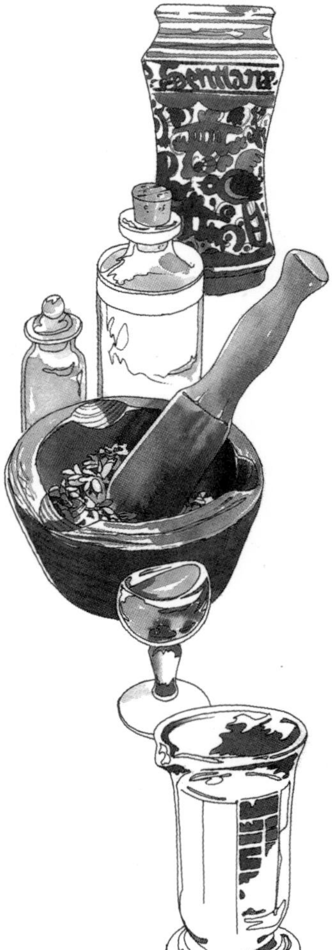

KAMPO MEDICATIONS AND THE FUTURE . . .

Once Kampo was fully established here in Japan, the firm of Tsumura became a leading supplier of the crude herbs needed by its practitioners. Working with them, our next step was to offer ready-mixed combinations of herbal remedies most often prescribed by doctors. By establishing a reputable and safe source of medicine, and making treatment easier for patient and doctor, Tsumura became the leading marketer of Kampo medicine in the world.

Now, we are ready for the "New Medicine" of the future. We have already exceeded all the strict requirements of the government's watchdog agencies. Quality control is hi-tech, carried out with the help of a computer monitoring system. From the raw plants to the final refined pharmaceutical product there are 3,000 check points to guarantee quality.

These Kampo medicines typically contain between four and eighteen different crude drug extracts. Experience shows that when a Kampo medicine is taken as treatment for a particular ailment the interaction, or synergy, of the crude drugs is far more significant than the specific reaction of each individual crude drug. This is perhaps the most miraculous of all the capacities of Kampo, that the medicines work so naturally and completely to restore total physical well being. In western idiom, they are "user friendly!"

In the following pages you will find the herbal formulas that have built Tsumura reputation in Japan and in Europe. According to plan, a carefully selected number will soon be available in the U.S. as well—perhaps only as over-the-counter drugs—because of the long time it will take to substantiate claims by law for each one of the remedies described in these pages. This long process is required of all drug firms in the U.S. However, if you wish to keep up with the progress we make in our laboratories, and in marketing Kampo in the U.S., please write us on a professional letterhead and we will add you to our overseas mailing list for medical literature. Write: Tsumura & Co., Tsuchiura, 12–7 Nibancho, Chiyoda-ku, Tokyo 102, Japan.

What next? In the decade of the '90s, we expect to add many more new herbal combinations based on research now going on regularly in all our scientific institutes using new techniques from molecular biology to chemical compound synthesis. In my own lifetime I expect to see the discovery of herbal drugs which will cure a good many of the tragic, frustrating illnesses still plaguing mankind.

Kakkon-to 葛根湯

• Efficacy

Used for those who do not perspire spontaneously and have headaches, fever, chills, stiff shoulders etc. with a relatively strong constitution accompanied with the following illnesses:

Common cold, nose cold, early stages of a febrile disease, inflammatory diseases (conjunctivitis, keratitis, tympanitis, tonsillitis, mastitis, lymphadenitis), stiff shoulders, neuralgia in the upper half of the body and urticaria.

• Ingredients

Puerariae Radix	4.0 g
Zizyphi Fructus	3.0 g
Ephedrae Herba	3.0 g
Glycyrrhizae Radix	2.0 g
Cinnamomi Cortex	2.0 g
Paeoniae Radix	2.0 g
Zingiberis Rhizoma	2.0 g

• Usage=SHO

This prescription is used for those with a relatively strong constitution during the early stages of an inflammatory disease, diseases accompanied with pain or during accute stages of a chronic disease.

1) Early stages of colds and other febrile diseases where there are chills, fever, headaches and stiff nape of the neck with no spontaneous perspiration.
2) Diseases accompanied with pain where there is local pain, swelling, redness etc.
3) The early stages of skin diseases where there is redness, swelling and severe irritation.

Otsuji-to 乙字湯

• Efficacy

Used when the illness is not so serious, average constitution, not weak, with the following complaints:

Hemorrhoids.

• Ingredients

Angelicae Radix	6.0 g
Bupleurae Radix	5.0 g
Scutellariae Radix	3.0 g

Glycyrrhizae Radix .... 2.0 g
Cimicifugae Rhizoma .... 1.0 g
Zizyphi Fructus .... 0.5 g

• Usage=SHO
Used for those who have an average constitution with hemorrhoids where the symptoms are not so severe.
1) Tendency to have constipation.
2) Pain and/or itchiness of the anus or genitals.
3) Light hemorrhaging.

Anchu-san 安中散

• Efficacy
Used for thin patients with a tendency to have a lack of tone of the abdominal muscles with stomach or abdominal pain, occasional heartburn, belching, loss of appetite, and nausea with the following illnesses:
Neurotic gastritis, chronic gastritits, stomach atony.

• Ingredients
Cinnamomi Cortex .... 4.0 g
Corydalis Tuber .... 3.0 g
Ostreae Testa .... 3.0 g
Foeniculi Fructus .... 1.5 g
Glycyrrhizae Radix .... 1.0 g
Amomi Semen .... 1.0 g
Alpiniae Officinarum Rhizoma .... 0.5 g

• Usage=SHO
Used for those who are thin and have a relatively weak constitution and have stomach pain and/or heartburn which has become chronic.
1) Bad digestion of food, a feeling of distention in the epigastrium, nausea, vomiting etc.
2) Soft weak abdomen with a splashing sound upon palpation in the epigastrium.

Hachimi-jio-gan 八味地黄丸

• Efficacy
Used for patients with fatigue, tiredness, oliguria or frequent urination, thirst and alternating coldness and hotness of the extremities with the following illnesses:

Nephritis, diabetes, impotence, sciatica, lumbago, beri-beri, urinary bladder catarrh, hypertrophy of the prostatic gland, hypertension.

• Ingredients

Rehmanniae Radix	6.0 g
Corni Fructus	3.0 g
Dioscoreae Rhizoma	3.0 g
Alismatis Rhizoma	3.0 g
Hoelen	3.0 g
Moutan Cortex	2.5 g
Cinnamomi Cortex	1.0 g
Processed Aconiti Tuber	0.5 g

• Usage=SHO

Often used for those in middle age and above, especially the elderly, who have lost strength; coldness and numbness of the lower back and legs and urinary irregularities (especially frequent urination at night).

1) In comparison to the upper abdomen the lower abdomen is soft, weak and powerless.
2) Polyuria, frequent urination, oliguria, dysuria etc.
3) Fatigue, lumbago, thirst etc.

Dai-saiko-to 大柴胡湯

• Efficacy

Used for those who have a relatively strong constitution with constipation, discomfort and distention of the upper abdomen, tinnitus and stiff shoulders accompanied with the following illnesses:

Gall stones, cholecystitis, jaundice, liver function disorders, hypertension, cerebral anemia, urticaria, gastric hyperacidity, acute gastroenteric catarrh, nausea, vomiting, loss of appetite, hemorrhoids, diabetes, neurosis, insomnia.

• Ingredients

Bupleuri Radix	6.0 g
Pinelliae Tuber	4.0 g
Scutellariae Radix	3.0 g
Paeoniae Radix	3.0 g
Zizyphi Fructus	3.0 g
Aurantii Fructus Immaturus	2.0 g
Zingiberis Rhizoma	1.0 g
Rhei Rhizoma	1.0 g

• Usage=SHO
Used for those with a strong build and constitution, severe tenderness and distention of the hypochondrium and constipation.
1) Nausea, vomiting, discomfort and distention of the hypochondrium etc.
2) Stiff shoulders, headache, head feels heavy, vertigo, tinnitus etc.

Sho-saiko-to 小柴胡湯

• Efficacy
Used for those with an average constitution who have discomfort and distention of the upper abdomen, tongue fur, unpleasant feeling in the mouth, loss of appetite, nausea, and may occasionally have low grade fever with the following illnesses:
Various febrile diseases, pneumonia, bronchitis, colds, pleurisy, tuberculosis, lymphangitis, chronic complaints of the digestive system, liver complaints, incomplete recovery from child-birth.

• Ingredients

Bupleuri Radix	7.0 g
Pinelliae Tuber	5.0 g
Scutellariae Radix	3.0 g
Zizyphi Fructus	3.0 g
Ginseng Radix	3.0 g
Glycyrrhizae Radix	2.0 g
Zingiberis Rhizoma	1.0 g

• Usage=SHO
Used for those with an average constitution with tenderness and distention of the hypochondrium.
1) Febrile diseases accompanied with a loss of appetite, unpleasant feeling in the mouth etc.
2) Various chronic diseases which are accompanied with tenderness and distention of the hypochondrium.
3) Various chronic diseases which are accompanied with loss of appetite, fatigue etc.
4) Strengthens children with weak constitutions.

Saiko-keishi-to 柴胡桂枝湯

• Efficacy
Used for those with fever accompanied by perspiration, chills, headaches and nausea with the following illnesses:

Common cold, influenza, pneumonia, pulmonary tuberculosis, gastric ulcers, duodenal ulcers, cholecystitis, liver function disorders, pancreatitis and other illnesses with tension and pain in the epigastrium.

• Ingredients

Bupleuri Radix	5.0 g
Pinelliae Tuber	4.0 g
Scutellariae Radix	2.0 g
Glycyrrhizae Radix	2.0 g
Cinnamomi Cortex	2.0 g
Paeoniae Radix	2.0 g
Zizyphi Fructus	2.0 g
Ginseng Radix	2.0 g
Zingiberis Rhizoma	1.0 g

• Usage=SHO

Used for febrile diseases which have passed through the acute stage accompanied with headaches, chills, joint pain, loss of appetite etc. In chronic diseases there is discomfort and distention in the epigastrium and hypochondrium with resistance and pain upon pressure (palpation) and cramps of the abdominus rectus (the muscles running vertically up the abdomen).

1) Discomfort and distention of the epigastrium, loss of appetite, abdominal pain etc.
2) Anxiety, insomnia and other psychoneurotic symptoms.

Saiko-keishi-kankyo-to 柴胡桂枝乾姜湯

• Efficacy

Used for those who have a weak, cold constitution with anemia, palpitations, shortness of breath and are high strung accompanied with the following illnesses:
Climacteric disorders, hysteria, neurosis, insomnia etc.

• Ingredients

Bupleuri Radix	6.0 g
Scutellariae Radix	3.0 g
Trichosanthis Radix	3.0 g
Cinnamomi Cortex	3.0 g
Ostreae Testa	3.0 g
Glycyrrhizae Radix	2.0 g
Zingiberis Siccatum Radix	2.0 g

• Usage=SHO

Used for those with a relatively weak constitution who have a pale complexion, fatigue, palpitations, shortness of breath, insomnia and other psychoneurotic symptoms.

1) Light discomfort and distention of the epigastrium and hypochondrium.
2) Chills, low grade fever, night sweat, thirst etc.

Saiko-ka-ryukotsu-borei-to 柴胡加竜骨牡蛎湯

• Efficacy

Used for those with a relatively strong constitution who have tachycardia, insomnia, irritability and other psychoneurotic symptoms with the following diseases:

Hypertension, arteriosclerosis, chronic kidney diseases, neurasthenia, neurotic tachycardia, epilepsy, hysteria, childrens' night crying, impotence.

• Ingredients

Bupleuri Radix	5.0 g
Pinelliae Tuber	4.0 g
Cinnamomi Cortex	3.0 g
Hoelen	3.0 g
Scutellariae Radix	2.5 g
Zizyphi Fructus	2.5 g
Ginseng Radix	2.5 g
Ostreae Testa	2.5 g
Fossilia Ossis Mastodi	2.5 g
Zigiberis Rhizoma	1.0 g

Usage=SHO

Used for those with a relatively strong constitution, mental anxiety, insomnia, irritability and other psychoneurotic symptoms with tenderness and distention of the hypochondrium.

1) Headaches, head feeling heavy, stiff shoulders etc.
2) A palpitation can be felt near the umbilicus on the abdomen when palpated.

Hange-shashin-to 半夏瀉心湯

• Efficacy

Used for those with discomfort of the epigastrium accompanied by occasional nausea or vomiting, loss of appetite, borborygmus and losse stools or diarrhea with the following diseases:

Acute or chronic gastroenteric catarrh, putrid diarrhea, indigestion, gastroptosis, neurotic gastritis, weak stomach, hangover, belching, heartburn, stomatitis, neurosis.

• Ingredients

Pinelliae Tuber	5.0 g
Scutellariae Radix	2.5 g
Glycyrrhizae Radix	2.5 g
Zizyphi Fructus	2.5 g
Ginseng Radix	2.5 g
Coptidis Rhizoma	1.0 g
Zingiberis Siccatum	2.5 g

• Usage=SHO

Used for those with an average constitution with a feeling of distention in the epigastrium, borborygmus, nausea, vomiting, diarrhea etc.

1) Loss of appetite, light pain in the upper abdomen etc.
2) Anxiety, insomnia and other psychoneurotic symptoms.

Oren-gedoku-to 黄連解毒湯

• Efficacy

Used for those with a relatively strong constitution who have head-rushes, and irritability with the following diseases:

Hemoptysis, hematemesis, blood in the stools, cerebral anemia, hypertension, tachycardia, neurosis, pruritis cutaneus (itchy skin), gastritis.

• Ingredients

Scutellariae Radix	3.0 g
Coptidis Rhizoma	2.0 g
Gardeniae Fructus	2.0 g
Phellodendri Cortex	1.5 g

Usage=SHO

Used for those who have an average to above average strength constitution with hot, red flushes of the face, mental anxiety, insomnia, irritability and other psychoneurotic symptoms.

1) The epigastrium feels distended.
2) Nose bleeds, coughing blood, vomiting blood, bleeding hemorrhoids, blood in the stool and other types of hemorrhaging.
3) Skin diseases with eruptions and itchiness.

Hange-koboku-to 半夏厚朴湯

• Efficacy

Used for those who feel depressed and have a feeling of something being stuck in the throat or esophagus, with occasional palpitations, vertigo and nausea accompanied with the following illnesses:

Anxiety, neurotic gastritis, morning sickness, coughing, hoarse voice, neurotic esophagostenosis, insomnia.

• Ingredients

Pinelliae Tuber	6.0 g
Hoelen	5.0 g
Magnoliae Cortex	3.0 g
Perillae Herba	2.0 g
Zingiberis Rhizoma	1.0 g

• Usage=SHO

Used for those with an average to below average constitution who have a pale complexion, neurotic tendencies and a blocked feeling in the throat (globus hystericus).

1) Depression, insomnia, palpitations and anxiety.
2) Breathing difficulties, coughing and pain in the chest.
3) Splashing sound in the epigastrium upon palpation.

Keishi-ka-jutsubu-to 桂枝加朮附湯

• Efficacy

Used for joint pain and neuralgia.

• Ingredients

Cinnamomi Cortex	4.0 g
Paeoniae Radix	4.0 g
Atractylodis Lanceae Rhizoma	4.0 g
Zizyphi Fructus	4.0 g
Glycyrrhizae Radix	2.0 g
Zingiberis Rhizoma	1.0 g
Processed and powdered Aconiti Tuber	0.5 g

• Usage=SHO

Used for those with a cold, weak constitution who have joint pain and swelling, muscle pain, movement impediments of the extremities etc.

1) Joint pain, muscle pain etc. which becomes worse with the cold.
2) Low grade fever, night sweat, stiffness of the hands in the morning and scanty urine.

Sho-seiryu-to 小青竜湯

• Efficacy

Used for bronchitis, bronchial asthma, watery nasal discharge, cough accompanied with watery expectoration, and rhinitis.

• Ingredients

Pinelliae Tuber	6.0 g
Glycyrrhizae Radix	3.0 g
Cinnamomi Cortex	3.0 g
Schisandrae Fructus	3.0 g
Asiasari Radix	3.0 g
Paeoniae Radix	3.0 g
Ephedrae Herba	3.0 g
Zingiberis Siccatum Rhizoma	3.0 g

• Usage=SHO

Used for those who have an average constitution with asthma, coughing, breathing difficulties, nasal symptoms etc.

1) Foam-like watery phlegm, watery nasal discharge, sneezing etc.
2) Splashing sound in the epigastrium upon palpation.

Boi-ogi-to 防已黄耆湯

• Efficacy

Used for those who have a white skin, soft muscles and fluid retention which causes overweight, tire easily, perspire a lot, and have dysuria with edema of the legs accompanied with the following illnesses:

Nephritis, nephosis, pregnancy kidney, scrotal hydrocele, obesity, joint inflammations, carbuncles, edema, skin diseases, over-perspiration, irregular menstruation.

• Ingredients

Astragali Radix	5.0 g
Sinomeni Caulis et Rhizoma	5.0 g
Atractylodis Lanceae Rhizoma	3.0 g

Zizyphi Fructus .... 3.0 g
Glycyrrhizae Radix .... 1.5 g
Zingiberis Rhizoma .... 1.0 g

• Usage=SHO
Used for those with a relatively weak constitution, white complexion, soft muscles, overweight with fluid, fatigue, and a tendency to perspire much.

1) Edema, scanty urine, swelling and pain of the joints (especially the knees).

Sho-hange-ka-bukuryo-to 小半夏加茯苓湯

• Efficacy
For those with an average constitution with the following illnesses:

Morning sickness and other illnesses accompanied by vomiting (acute gastro-enteritis, wet pleurisy, beri beri with edema, empyema).

• Ingredients
Pinelliae Tuber .... 6.0 g
Hoelen .... 5.0 g
Zingiberis Rhizoma .... 1.5 g

• Usage=SHO
Used for those with an average constitution with nausea and vomiting.

1) Vomit a small amount at a time; after vomiting are still left with nausea.
2) Discomfort in the epigastrium, vertigo, palpitations etc.

Toki-shakuyaku-san 当帰芍薬散

• Efficacy
Used for those with soft muscles who tire easily and have cold legs and lower back accompanied with the following illnesses:

Anemia, fatigue, climacteric disorders (heavy head, headache, vertigo, stiff shoulders etc.), irregular menstruation, dysmenorrhea, infertility, palpitations, chronic nephritis, various symptoms which appear due to pregnancy (edema, habitual abortion, hemorrhoids, abdominal pain), beri beri, hemiplegia, valvular heart disease.

• Ingredients
Paeoniae Radix .... 4.0 g

Atractylodis Lanceae Rhizoma .... 4.0 g
Alismatis Rhizoma .... 4.0 g
Hoelen .... 4.0 g
Cnidii Rhizoma .... 3.0 g
Angelicae Radix .... 3.0 g

- Usage=SHO

This prescription is often used for adult women with a relatively weak constitution. In general, they feel the cold easily and tend to have anemia, light edema around and during menstruation period, and abdominal pain.

1) Fatigue, cold extremities, headaches, vertigo, tinnitus, stiff shoulders, tachycardia, etc.
2) No menstruation, copious menstruation, menstrual difficulties and other menstrual irregularities.
3) Various symptoms which occur during pregnancy or after childbirth.

Kami-shoyo-san 加味逍遙散

- Efficacy

Used for women with weak constitutions who have stiff shoulders, tire easily, and have anxiety and other psychoneurotic symptoms (they may also tend to get constipation), accompanied with the following illnesses:

Cold constitution, weak constitution, irregular menstruation, dismenorrhea, climacteric disorders, neurosis etc.

- Ingredients

Bupleuri Radix .... 3.0 g
Paeoniae Radix .... 3.0 g
Atractylodis Lancea Rhizoma .... 3.0 g
Angelicae Radix .... 3.0 g
Hoelen .... 3.0 g
Gargeniae Fructus .... 2.0 g
Moutan Cortex .... 2.0 g
Glycyrrhizae Radix .... 1.5 g
Zingiberis Rhizoma .... 1.0 g
Menthae Herba .... 1.0 g

- Usage=SHO

Used for those with a relatively weak constitution who tire easily and suffer from mental anxiety, insomnia, irritability and other psychoneurotic conditions.

1) Stiff shoulders, headaches, vertigo, hot flushes in the upper body and attack-like bouts of perspiration etc.

2) Light tenderness and resistance upon palpation of the epigastrium and hypochondrium.
3) Psychoneurotic symptoms which occur near menstruation (PMS).

Keishi-bukuryo-gan 桂枝茯苓丸

• Efficacy

Used for those with a strong constitution, these patients also often have a ruddy complexion, the abdomen wall is strong and there is resistance in the lower abdomen accompanied with the following illnesses:

Inflammation of the uterus or other related organs, endometritis, irregular menstruation, dysmenorrhea, leukorrhea, climacteric disorders (headaches, vertigo, flushes, stiff shoulders etc.), cold constitution, peritonitis, bruising, hemorrhoids, orchitis.

• Ingredients

Cinnamomi Cortex	3.0 g
Paeoniae Radix	3.0 g
Persicae Semen	3.0 g
Hoelen	3.0 g
Moutan Cortex	3.0 g

• Usage=SHO

Used for those with an above average strength constitution who often have flushes and a ruddy complexion; there is resistance and pain upon pressure in the lower abdomen. It is used for conditions accompanying blood stagnation.

1) Headaches, stiff shoulders, vertigo, flushes, cold feet/legs etc.
2) Amenorrhea, hypermenorrhea, dysmenorrhea and other menstrual disorders in women.

Mao-to 麻黄湯

• Efficacy

Used for those suffering from chills, fever, headaches, lower-back pain and no spontaneous perspiration with the following illnesses:

Colds, influenza (early stages), rheumatoid arthritis, asthma, infant's nasal blockage, infants who have difficulty suckling.

● Ingredients

Armeniacae Semen	5.0 g
Ephedra Herba	5.0 g
Cinnamomi Cortex	4.0 g
Glycyrrhizae Radix	1.5 g

● Usage=SHO

Used for those who normally have a strong constitution and during the early stages of febrile diseases. Patients have headaches, fever, chills, lower-back pain and pain in the joints. They do not have any spontaneous perspiration.

1) Asthma, coughing etc.
2) Common cold in infants accompanied with nasal blockage.

Bakumondo-to 麦門冬湯

● Efficacy

Cough with difficult-to-expel phlegm, bronchitis, bronchial asthma.

● Ingredients

Ophiopogonis Tuber	10.0 g
Pinelliae Tuber	5.0 g
Zizyphi Fructus	3.0 g
Glycyrrhizae Radix	2.0 g
Ginseng Radix	2.0 g
Oryzae Fructus	5.0 g

● Usage=SHO

Used for those who have an average to weaker than average constitution with a severe cough which comes in attacks and causes the face to become red.

1) Very difficult to bring up phlegm.
2) A dryness or discomfort in the throat.
3) Cough in pregnant women or elderly people.

Shimbu-to 真武湯

● Efficacy

For those whose metabolism has become severely weakened with the following illnesses:

Gastrointestinal disorders, weak digestive system, chronic enteritis, indigestion, stomach atony, gastroptosis, nephrosis, peritonitis, cerebral anemia, paralysis and/ or movement impediments due to illnesses of the spinal cord, weak nerves, hypertension, valvular heart disease, cardiac insufficiency with tachycardia, hemiplegia, rheumatoid arthritis, geriatric itchiness.

• Ingredients

Hoelen	4.0 g
Paeoniae Radix	3.0 g
Atractylodis Lanceas Rhizoma	3.0 g
Zingiberis Rhizoma	1.5 g
Processed Aconiti Tuber	0.5 g

• Usage=SHO

Used for those whose metabolism has become severely weak and have a weak constitution, general fatigue, coldness of the extremities, diarrhea, abdominal pain etc.

1) The diarrhea for which this formula is prescribed is not accompanied with abdominal cramps.
2) Vertigo, trembling, tachycardia etc.

Ninjin-to 人参湯

• Efficacy

Used for those who have a weak constitution with the following illnesses:

Acute and chronic gastroenteric catarrh, stomach atony, gastrodilation, morning sickness, nephrosclerosis.

• Ingredients

Glycyrrhizae Radix	3.0 g
Atractylodis Lancea Radix	3.0 g
Ginseng Radix	3.0 g
Zingiberis Siccatum Rhizoma	3.0 g

• Usage=SHO

Used for those who have a relatively weak and cold constitution with loss of appetite, a feeling of stagnancy in the stomach area, diarrhea and other digestive system functional weaknesses.

1) Weak digestive system, fatigue, copious lightly coloured urine, much thin saliva in the mouth etc.
2) A soft weak abdominal wall with a splash upon palpitation in the epigastrium.

Daio-botampi-to 大黄牡丹皮湯

• Efficacy

Used for those who have a relatively strong constitution with pain in the lower abdomen and constipation with any of the following illnesses:

Irregular menstruation, dysmenorrhea, constipation, hemorrhoids.

• Ingredients

Persicae Semen	4.0 g
Moutan Cortex	4.0 g
Rhei Rhizoma	2.0 g
Benincasae Semen	6.0 g
Natrium Sulfuricum	1.8 g

• Usage=SHO

Used for those who have a relatively strong constitution with tension, resistance and pain in the lower abdomen, constipation and blood stagnation.

1) Dysmenorrhea, copious menstruation, and other menstrual irregularities.

Byakko-ka-ninjin-to 白虎加人参湯

• Efficacy

Used for those who have thirst and hotness of the body.

• Ingredients

Gypsum Fibrosum	15.0 g
Anemarrhenae Rhizoma	5.0 g
Glycyrrhizae Radix	2.0 g
Ginseng Radix	1.5 g
Oryzae Fructus	8.0 g

• Usage=SHO

Used for those with a relatively strong constitution with general hotness of the body, thirst, and much urine.

1) Skin diseases with severe irritation (itching).

Shigyaku-san 四逆散

• Efficacy

Used for those with a relatively strong constitution who are between Dai-saiko-to-sho and Sho-saiko-to-sho with any of the following illnesses:

Cholecyctitis, gall stones, gastritis, gastric hyperacidity, gastric ulcers, nasal catarrh, bronchitis, nervousness, hysteria.

• Ingredients

Bupleuri Radix	5.0 g
Paeoniae Radix	4.0 g
Aurantii Fructus Immaturus	2.0 g
Glycyrrhizae Radix	1.5 g

• Usage=SHO

Used for those with an average to strong constitution with tenderness upon palpation and distention of the hypochondrium, abdominal muscle cramps, irritability, insomnia, depression and other psychoneurotic symptoms.

1) Abdominal pain, a feeling of distention in the abdomen, palpitations etc.

Moku-boi-to 木防已湯

• Efficacy

Used for those who have a pale complexion, breathing difficulties with coughing, heart or kidney diseases accompanied with a feeling of tension and heaviness below the heart (epigastrium), edema and cardiac asthma.

• Ingredients

Gypsum Fibrosum	10.0 g
Sinomeni Caulis et Rhizoma	4.0 g
Cinnamomi Cortex	3.0 g
Ginseng Radix	3.0 g

• Usage=SHO

Used for those with a relatively weak constitution who have discomfort and hardness of the epigastrium, breathing difficulties, edema and palpitations etc.

1) Thirst, scanty urine etc.

Ryo-kei-jutsu-kan-to 苓桂朮甘湯

• Efficacy

Used for those with vertigo, faintness, palpitations, and scanty urine with any of the following illnesses:

Nervousness, neurosis, vertigo, palpitations, shortness of breath, headaches.

• Ingredients

Hoelen	6.0 g
Cinnamomi Cortex	4.0 g
Atractylodis Lancea Rhizoma	3.0 g
Glycyrrhizae Radix	2.0 g

• Usage=SHO

Used for those with a relatively weak constitution, vertigo, a feeling of the body trembling, dizziness upon standing etc.

1) Shortness of breath, tachycardia, headaches, headrushes, scanty urine etc.
2) A splash in the epigastrium upon palpation.

Chorei-to 猪苓湯

• Efficacy

Scanty urine, dysuria, thirst with any of the following illnesses:

Urethritis, nephritis, kidney stones, gonorrhea, pain upon urination, hematuria, edema from the waist down, incomplete urination, diarrhea.

• Ingredients

Alismatis Rhizoma	3.0 g
Polyporus	3.0 g
Hoelen	3.0 g
Asini Gelatinum	3.0 g
Kadinum	3.0 g

• Usage=SHO

Without any consideration for the constitution, it is used to treat polyuria, incomplete urination, dysuria, hematuria and other urinary disorders.

Hochu-ekki-to 補中益気湯

• Efficacy

Weakened digestive function, tired extremities, and a weak constitution with any of the following illnesses:

Weight loss in summer, weakness after illness, tuberculosis, loss of appetite, gastroptosis, colds, hemorrhoids, prolapsed rectum, prolapsed uterus, impotence, hemiplegia, copious perspiration.

• Ingredients

Astragali Radix	4.0 g
Atractylodis Lancea Rhizoma	4.0 g
Ginseng Radix	4.0 g
Angelicae Radix	3.0 g
Bupleuri Radix	2.0 g
Zizyphi Fructus	2.0 g
Aurantii Nobilis Pericarpium	2.0 g
Glycyrrhizae Radix	1.5 g
Cimicifugae Rhizoma	1.0 g
Zingiberis Rhizoma	0.5 g

• Usage=SHO

Used for those who have a relatively weak constitution who suffer from fatigue, loss of appetite etc.

1) Weak constitution with tuberculosis or other chronic conditions.
2) Convalescing after operations or illness, post-partum conditions etc.
3) Coughing, low grade fever, night sweat, palpitations etc.

Rikkunshi-to 六君子湯

• Efficacy

A weak digestive system with loss of appetite, discomfort in the epigastrium, tires easily, anemic and cold extremities accompaning any of the following illnesses:

Gastritis, gastric atony, gastroptosis, indigestion, loss of appetite, stomach ache, vomiting.

• Ingredients

Atractylodis Lancea Rhizoma	4.0 g
Ginseng Radix	4.0 g
Pinelliae Tuber	4.0 g
Hoelen	4.0 g
Zizyphi Fructus	2.0 g

Aurantii Nobilis Pericarpium .... 2.0 g
Glycyrrhizae Radix .... 1.0 g
Zingiberis Rhizoma .... 0.5 g

● Usage=SHO

Used for those who have a relatively weak constitution and digestive system function with a loss of appetite, a feeling of distention in the epigastrium etc.

1) General fatigue, cold extremities etc.
2) A weak abdominal wall and a splash in the epigastrium upon palpation.

Keishi-to 桂枝湯

● Efficacy

Used for those with a weak constitution in the early stages of colds.

● Ingredients

Cinnamomi Cortex .... 4.0 g
Paeoniae Radix .... 4.0 g
Zizyphi Fructus .... 4.0 g
Glycyrrhizae Radix .... 2.0 g
Zingiberis Rhizoma .... 1.5 g

● Usage=SHO

Used for those who have a relatively weak constitution with headaches, fever, chills, general pain in the body and spontaneous perspiration.

Shichimotsu-koka-to 七物降下湯

● Efficacy

For those who tend to have a weak constitution with any of the following illnesses:

Hypertension with associated symptoms (headrushes, stiff shoulders, tinnitus, heavy head).

● Ingredients

Paeoniae Radix .... 4.0 g
Angelicae Radix .... 4.0 g
Astragli Radix .... 3.0 g
Rehmanniae Radix .... 3.0 g
Cnidii Rhizoma .... 3.0 g
Phellodendri Cortex .... 2.0 g
Uncariae Ramulus et Uncus .... 3.0 g

● Usage=SHO
Used for those with a weak constitution but have a relatively strong digestive system with hypertension.
1) Easily become fatigued, coldness of the lower body, tendency to have frequent urination.

Choto-san 釣藤散

● Efficacy
For those middle aged and under with continuous chronic headache and for those with a tendency to have hypertension.

● Ingredients

Gypsum Fibrosum	5.0 g
Aurantii Nobilis Pericarpium	3.0 g
Ophiopogonis Tuber	3.0 g
Pinelliae Tuber	3.0 g
Hoelen	3.0 g
Ginseng Radix	2.0 g
Ledebouriellae Radix	2.0 g
Glycyrrhizae Radix	1.0 g
Zingiberis Rhizoma	1.0 g
Uncariae Ramulus et Uncus	3.0 g
Chrysanthemi Flos	2.0 g

● Usage=SHO
Used for those with an average constitution or those middle aged and under with a slightly weakened constitution who have headaches which have become chronic, stiff shoulders, vertigo etc.
1) There is a tendency to get headaches or a heaviness of the head upon waking in the morning.
2) Headrushes, tinnitus, insomnia, blood congestion of the cornea etc.

Juzen-taiho-to 十全大補湯

● Efficacy
Used for weakened conditions after illness, fatigue, loss of appetite, night sweat, cold extremities, anemia.

• Ingredients

Astragali Radix	3.0 g
Cinnamomi Cortex	3.0 g
Rehmanniae Radix	3.0 g
Paeoniae Radix	3.0 g
Cnidii Rhizoma	3.0 g
Atractylodis Lancea Rhizoma	3.0 g
Angelicae Radix	3.0 g
Ginseng Radix	3.0 g
Hoelen	3.0 g
Glycyrrhizae Radix	1.5 g

• Usage=SHO

Used for those who are in a weakened condition due to illness or surgery etc.

1) General fatigue, loss of appetite, pale complexion, dry skin, anemia etc.
2) Night sweat, dryness of the mouth etc.

Sokei-kakketsu-to 疎経活血湯

• Efficacy

Joint pain, neuralgia, muscle pain.

• Ingredients

Paeoniae Radix	2.5 g
Rehmanniae Radix	2.0 g
Cnidii Rhizoma	2.0 g
Atractylodis Lancea Rhizoma	2.0 g
Angelicae Radix	2.0 g
Persicae Semen	2.0 g
Hoelen	2.0 g
Achyranthis Radix	1.5 g
Aurantii Nobilis Pericarpium	1.5 g
Sinomeni Caulis et Rhizoma	1.5 g
Ledebouriellae Radix	1.5 g
Gentianae Scabrae Radix	1.5 g
Glycyrrhizae Radix	1.0 g
Angelicae Dahuricae Radix	1.0 g
Zingiberis Rhizoma	0.5 g
Clemantidis Radix	1.5 g
Notopterygii Rhizoma	1.5 g

• Usage=SHO

Used for those with an average constitution with muscle, joint and nerve pain in the area from the lower back down to the legs.

1) Often becomes worse when cold.
2) Accompanied with blood stagnation.

Ma-kyo-kan-seki-to 麻杏甘石湯

• Efficacy

Children's asthma, bronchial asthma.

• Ingredients

Gypsum Fibrosum .... 10.0 g
Armeniacae Semen .... 4.0 g
Ephedrae Herba .... 4.0 g
Glycyrrhizae Radix .... 2.0 g

• Usage=SHO

It is used for those who have a relatively strong constitution with severe coughing, thirst, spontaneous perspiration, fever, stridor and breathing difficulties.

1) Sticky phlegm which is often difficult to expel.
2) Often used for children.

Gorin-san 五淋散

• Efficacy

Frequent urination, dysuria, feeling of incomplete urination.

• Ingredients

Hoelen .... 6.0 g
Scutellariae Radix .... 3.0 g
Glycyrrhizae Radix .... 3.0 g
Rehmanniae Radix .... 3.0 g
Plantaginis Semen .... 3.0 g
Alismatis Rhizoma .... 3.0 g
Angelicae Radix .... 3.0 g
Akebiae Caulis .... 3.0 g
Gardeniae Fructus .... 2.0 g
Paeoniae Radix .... 2.0 g
Kadinum .... 3.0 g

• Usage=SHO

Used for those with an average to weak constitution who have chronic urethritis accompanied with frequent urination, a feeling of incomplete urination, dysuria etc.

Unsei-in 温清飲

• Efficacy

Used for those who have lack-lustre skin and headrushes with the following illnesses:

Irregular menstration, amenorrhea, hysteria, climacteric disorders, neurosis.

• Ingredients

Rehmanniae Radix	3.0 g
Paeoniae Radix	3.0 g
Cnidii Rhizoma	3.0 g
Angelicae Radix	3.0 g
Scutellariae Radix	1.5 g
Phellodendri Cortex	1.5 g
Coptidis Rhizoma	1.5 g
Gardeniae Fructus	1.5 g

• Usage=SHO

Used for those with an average constitution who have anxiety, insomnia, headrushes and other psychoneurotic symptoms accompanied with hemorrhaging tendencies.

1) The skin is often a yellow-brown color and dry.
2) Blood in the stool, uterine hemorrhaging and menorrhagia (profuse menstruation).
3) Skin diseases where there is little secretion, redness, hotness and severe itchiness of the affected area.

Keishi-ka-shakuyaku-to 桂枝加芍薬湯

• Efficacy

Used for when the abdomen is distended with the following symptoms:

Gripe, abdominal pain.

• Ingredients

Paeoniae Radix	6.0 g

Cinnamomi Cortex .... 4.0 g
Zizyphi Fructus .... 4.0 g
Glycyrrhizae Radix .... 2.0 g
Zingiberis Rhizoma .... 1.0 g

• Usage=SHO
Used for those who have a relatively weak constitution with diarrhea or constipation accompanied with a distended abdomen, abdominal pain and tenesmus. This prescription is appropriate for those who have less severe tenesmus and constipation than keishi-ka-shakuyaku-daio-to-sho.

1) Although they feel like passing stools defecation does not occur.
2) Abdominal pain after using laxatives.
3) Difficulty in defecating after abdominal surgery.

Tokaku-joki-to 桃核承気湯

• Efficacy
Used for those who have a relatively strong constitution with headrushes and constipation accompanied with the following illnesses:

Irregular menstruation, amenorrhea, mental anxiety during menstruation or after child-birth, lumbago, constipation, symptoms accompanying hypertension (headache, vertigo, stiff shoulders).

• Ingredients
Persicae Semen .... 5.0 g
Cinnamomi Cortex .... 4.0 g
Rhei Rhizoma .... 3.0 g
Glycyrrhizae Radix .... 1.5 g
Natrium Sulfiuricum .... 0.9 g

• Usage=SHO
Used for those who have a strong constitution and blood stagnation with resistance and pain upon pressure in the lower left abdomen, constipation and headrushes.

1) Headaches, vertigo, insomnia, cold extremities and other psychoneurotic symptoms.
2) Irregular menstruation, dysmenorrhea etc.

Bofu-tsusho-san 防風通聖散

• Efficacy

Used for those with a thick layer of fat on the abdomen and constipation accompanied with the following illnesses:

Symptoms accompanying hypertension (palpitations, stiff shoulders, headrushes), obesity, edema, constipation.

• Ingredients

Scutellariae Radix	2.0 g
Glycyrrhizae Radix	2.0 g
Platycodi Radix	2.0 g
Gypsum Fibrosum	2.0 g
Atractylodis Rhizoma	2.0 g
Rhei Rhizoma	1.5 g
Schizonepetae Spica	1.2 g
Gardeniae Fructus	1.2 g
Paeoniae Radix	1.2 g
Cnidii Rhizoma	1.2 g
Angelicae Radix	1.2 g
Menthae Herba	1.2 g
Ledebouriellae Radix	1.2 g
Ephedrae Herba	1.2 g
Forsythiae Fructus	1.2 g
Zingiberis Rhizoma	0.3 g
Kadinum	3.0 g
Natrium Sulfuricum	0.7 g

• Usage=SHO

Used for those who have a strong constitution and a predisposition to having constipation, a strong, distended abdomen and a so-called "pot belly".

Sha-kanzo-to 炙甘草湯

• Efficacy

Used for those in weakened condition with fatigue, palpitations and shortness of breath.

• Ingredients

Rehmenniae Radix	6.0 g
Ophiopogonis Tuber	6.0 g
Cinnamomi Cortex	3.0 g

Zizyphi Fructus	3.0 g
Ginseng Radix	3.0 g
Zingiberis Rhizoma	1.0 g
Cannabidis Semen	3.0 g
Glycyrrhizae Radix (parched)	3.0 g
Asini Gelitinum	2.0 g

• Usage=SHO

Used for those who have a relatively weak constitution with palpitations and shortness of breath.

1) Dry skin, fatigue, hotness of the hands and feet.

Nyoshin-san 女神散

• Efficacy

Used for those who have head rushes and vertigo with the following illnesses: Pre/post-natal neurosis, irregular menstruation, hysteria.

• Ingredients

Cyperis Rhizoma	3.0 g
Cnidii Rhizoma	3.0 g
Atractylodis Rhizoma	3.0 g
Angelicae Radix	3.0 g
Scutellarae Radix	2.0 g
Cinnamomi Cortex	2.0 g
Ginseng Radix	2.0 g
Arecae Semen	2.0 g
Coptidis Rhizoma	1.0 g
Glycyrrhizae Radix	1.0 g
Caryophilli Flos	1.0 g
Saussureae Radix	1.0 g

• Usage=SHO

Used for those who have an average to strong constitution with headrushes, vertigo, anxiety, palpitations, insomnia, headaches and other psychoneurotic symptoms.

1) Various chronic complaints.
2) Symptoms accompanying menstruation or post-partum conditions.

Shikunshi-to 四君子湯

• Efficacy

Used for those who are thin and have a pale complexion, a loss of appetite and fatigue accompanying the following illnesses:

Weak digestive system, chronic gastritis, indigestion, vomiting, diarrhea.

• Ingredients

Atractylodis Lancea Rhizoma	4.0 g
Ginseng Radix	4.0 g
Hoelen	4.0 g
Glycyrrhizae Radix	1.0 g
Zingiberis Rhizoma	1.0 g
Zipyphi Fructus	1.0 g

• Usage=SHO

Used for those who have a weak constitution and digestive function with a loss of appetite, a feeling of distention in the abdomen etc.

1) The constitution is weaker than that for Rikkunshi-to-sho.
2) General fatigue, coldness of the extremities etc.
3) Weak abdominal muscles, a splashing sound can be heard in the epigastrium upon palpation.

Ryutan-shakan-to 竜胆瀉肝湯

• Efficacy

Used for those who have a relatively strong constitution with a tendency to have tense lower abdominal muscles accompanying the following illnesses:

Dysuria, a feeling of incomplete urination, urinary incontinence, leukorrhea.

• Ingredients

Rehmanniae Radix	5.0 g
Angelicae Radix	5.0 g
Akebiae Caulis	5.0 g
Scutellariae Radix	3.0 g
Plantaginis Semen	3.0 g
Alismatis Rhizoma	3.0 g
Glycyrrhizae Radix	1.0 g
Gardeniae Fructus	1.0 g
Gentianae Scabrae Radix	1.0 g

• Usage=SHO
Used for those who have a relatively strong constitution and inflammations of the urogenital organs with dysuria, frequent urination, leukorrhea etc.
1) Acute or chronic inflammations.
2) Itchiness of the sexual organs.

Kyuki-kyogai-to 芎帰膠艾湯

• Efficacy
Bleeding hemorrhoids

• Ingredients

Rehmanniae Radix	5.0 g
Paeoniae Radix	4.0 g
Angelicae Radix	4.0 g
Glycyrrhizae Radix	3.0 g
Cnidii Rhizoma	3.0 g
Artemisiae Folium	3.0 g
Asini Gelatinum	3.0 g

• Usage=SHO
Used for those who have a relatively weak constitution with hemorrhoids, blood in the stools, hemorrhaging of the urinary tract, irregular uterine hemorrhaging etc.
1) Continuous hemorrhaging with anemia, vertigo, cold extremities etc.

Yoku-kan-san-ka-chimpi-hange 抑肝散加陳皮半夏

• Efficacy
Used for those who have a weak constitution with a nervous temperament (high strung) accompanied with the following illnesses:
Neurosis, insomnia, children who cry at night, children's diseases.

• Ingredients

Pinelliae Tuber	5.0 g
Atractylodis Lancea Rhizoma	4.0 g
Hoelen	4.0 g
Cnidii Rhizoma	3.0 g
Aurantii Nobilis Pericarpium	3.0 g
Angelicae Radix	3.0 g

Bupleuri Radix	2.0 g
Glycyrrhizae Radix	1.5 g
Uncariae Ramulus et Uncus	3.0 g

• Usage=SHO

Used for those who have a relatively weak constitution who are easily excited, short tempered, irritable, and have insomnia and other psychoneurotic symptoms.

1) Children who are unsettled, have cramps and cry at night.
2) Spasms of the eyelids, trembling extremities etc.
3) Tense abdominus rectus.

Chikujo-untan-to 竹茹温胆湯

• Efficacy

Used during the recovery of influenza, common cold, pneumonia etc. where there is a continuous fever, or even though there may be no fever the patient suffers from general malaise, and due to coughing and/or much phlegm: he cannot sleep.

• Ingredients

Pinelliae Tuber	5.0 g
Bupleuri Radix	3.0 g
Ophiopogonis Tuber	3.0 g
Hoelen	3.0 g
Platycodi Radix	2.0 g
Aurantii Fructus Immaturus	2.0 g
Cyperi Rhizoma	2.0 g
Aurantii Nobilis Pericarpium	2.0 g
Coptidis Rhizoma	1.0 g
Glycyrrhizae Radix	1.0 g
Zingiberis Rhizoma	1.0 g
Ginseng Radix	1.0 g
Phyllostachysis Caulis in Taeniam	3.0 g

• Usage=SHO

Used for those who have a relatively weak constitution with a fever and/or coughing with phlegm and insomnia after a cold.

1) Mental anxiety, tachycardia etc.
2) Tenderness and resistance of the hypochondrium.

Sho-kenchu-to 小建中湯

• Efficacy

Used for those who have a weak constitution and tire easily with a pale complexion, abdominal pain, palpitations, hotness of the hands and feet, coldness, frequent or copious urine accompanied with the following illnesses:

Children with a weak constitution, fatigue, nervousness, chronic gastroenteritis, childrens nocturia/crying at night.

• Ingredients

Paeoniae Radix	6.0 g
Cinnamomi Cortex	4.0 g
Ziziphi Fructus	4.0 g
Glycyrrhizae Radix	2.0 g
Zingiberis Rhizoma	1.0 g

• Usage=SHO

Used for those who have a weak constitution and tire easily with a thin abdominal wall and tense abdominus rectus.

1) Abdominal pain.
2) Tachycardia, night sweat, nose bleeds, tired extremities etc.
3) Frequently used to strengthen children with weak constitutions.

Toki-to 当帰湯

• Efficacy

Used for those who have coldness of the back, distended feeling of the abdomen and abdominal pain.

• Ingredients

Angelicae Radix	5.0 g
Pinelliae Radix	5.0 g
Cinnamomi Cortex	3.0 g
Magnoliae Cortex	3.0 g
Paeoniae Radix	3.0 g
Ginseng Radix	3.0 g
Astragali Radix	1.5 g
Zanthoxyli Fructus	1.5 g
Glycyrrhizae Radix	1.0 g
Zingiberis Siccatum Rhizoma	1.5 g

• Usage=SHO
Cold, relatively weak constitution and a pale complexion with pain in the chest, abdomen and back.
1) Used for angina and intercostal neuralgia-like pain.

Unkeito 温経湯

• Efficacy
Used for those who have hotness of the hands and feet with dry lips accompanied with the following illnesses:
Irregular menstruation, amenorrhea, leukorrhea, climacteric disorders, insomnia, eczema, cold legs and lower back, frostbite.

• Ingredients

Ophiopogonis Tuber	4.0 g
Pinelliae Tuber	4.0 g
Angelicae Radix	3.0 g
Glycyrrhizae Radix	2.0 g
Cinnamomi Cortex	2.0 g
Pseoniae Radix	2.0 g
Cnidii Rhizoma	2.0 g
Ginseng Radix	2.0 g
Moutan Cortex	2.0 g
Evodiae Fructus	1.0 g
Zingiberis Rhizoma	1.0 g
Asini Gelatinum	2.0 g

• Usage=SHO
Used for those who have a relatively weak, cold constitution with hotness of the palms of the hands, dry lips, a cold, painful lower abdomen etc.
1) Hemorrhaging of the sexual organs, menstrual irregularities, infertility etc.
2) The above symptoms often become stronger or weaker around the time of menstruation.

Gosha-jinki-gan 牛車腎気丸

• Efficacy
Tire easily, cold extremities, scanty urine or copius urine with thirst accompanied with the following illnesses:

Leg pain, lumbago, numbness, geriatric cloudy vision, itchiness, pain upon urination, frequent urination, edema.

• Ingredients

Rehmanniae Radix	5.0 g
Achyranthis Radix	3.0 g
Corni Fructus	3.0 g
Dioscoreae Rhizoma	3.0 g
Plantaginis Semen	3.0 g
Alismatis Rhizoma	3.0 g
Hoelen	3.0 g
Moutan Cortex	3.0 g
Cinnamomi Cortex	1.0 g
Processed Aconiti Tuber	1.0 g

• Usage=SHO

Used for those who have a relatively weak constitution or elderly people with a loss of strength, coldness or numbness of the lower back and legs and urinary irregularities (especially frequent urination at night).

1) The symptoms are more pronounced than those of Hachimi-jio-gan-Sho.
2) The lower abdomen is soft in comparison to the upper abdomen.
3) Copious urine, frequent urination, oliguria, pain upon urination etc.
4) Fatigue, lumbago, thirst etc.

Seishin-renshi-in 清心蓮子飲

• Efficacy

General fatigue, dry mouth/tongue and urinary difficulties with the following illnesses:

Feeling of incomplete urination, frequent urination, pain upon urination.

• Ingredients

Ophiopogonis Tuber	4.0 g
Hoelen	4.0 g
Scutellariae Radix	3.0 g
Plataginis Semen	3.0 g
Ginseng Radix	3.0 g
Astragali Radix	2.0 g
Glycyrrhizae Radix	1.5 g
Nelumbinis Semen	4.0 g
Lycii Radicis Cortex	2.0 g

• Usago=SHO

Used for those who normally have a weak digestive system and constitution with olyguria, a feeling of incomplete urination, dysuria etc.

1) Often have a cold constitution and are nervous.
2) Chronic urogenital diseases.

Chorei-to-go-shimotsu-to 猪苓湯合四物湯

• Efficacy

Used for those who have dry skin, a lack-lustre, pale complexion and no digestive system problems accompanied with the following illnesses:

Olyguria, dysuria, a feeling of incomplete urination, frequent urination.

• Ingredients

Rehmanniae Radix	3.0 g
Paeoniae Radix	3.0 g
Cnidii Rhizoma	3.0 g
Alismatis Rhizoma	3.0 g
Polyporus	3.0 g
Angelicae Radix	3.0 g
Hoelen	3.0 g
Asini Gelatinum	3.0 g
Kadinum	3.0 g

• Usage=SHO

Used for those who have an average constitution with frequent urination, a feeling of incomplete urination, dysuria, hematuria and other urinary disorders which have become chronic or frequently occur.

San'o-shashin-to 三黄瀉心湯

• Efficacy

Used for those who have a relatively strong constitution with headrushes, flushes of the face, mental anxiety and constipation accompanied with the following illnesses:

Accompanying symptoms of hypertension (headrushes, stiff shoulders, tinnitus, heavy feeling of the head, insomnia, anxiety), nose bleeds, bleeding hemorrhoids, constipation, climacteric disorders, hysteria.

• Ingredients

Scutellariae Radix	3.0 g
Coptidis Rhizoma	3.0 g
Rhei Rhizoma	3.0 g

• Usage=SHO

Used for those who have a strong build and constitution with headrushes, flushes of the face and constipation.

1) Irritability, unsettled emotionally, anxiety and insomnia.
2) A feeling of distention in the epigastrium.
3) Nose bleeds, hemoptysis, hematosis, blood in the stools and other hemorrhaging signs. It should not be used when there has been continuous hemorrhaging and the patient is suffering from anemia.

Ryo-kyo-jutsu-kan-to 苓姜朮甘湯

• Efficacy

Used for those who have coldness and pain of the lower back and polyuria accompanied with the following illnesses:

Lumbago, cold lower back, nocturia.

• Ingredients

Hoelen	6.0 g
Atractylodis Rhizoma	3.0 g
Glycyrrhizae Radix	2.0 g
Zingiberis Siccatum Rhizoma	3.0 g

• Usage=SHO

Used for those who have a relatively weak constitution with coldness from the lower back to the legs and frequent urination.

1) Pain of the lower back and legs due to coldness.

Keishi-ka-shakuyaku-daio-to 桂枝加芍薬大黄湯

• Efficacy

Used for those who have a relatively weak constitution with a distended abdomen, a feeling of stagnation in the intestines or abdominal pain accompanied with the following illnesses:

1. Acute enteritis, catarrh of the large intestine.
2. Habitual constipation, retained stools, retching abdominal pain.

• Ingredients

Paeoniae Radix	6.0 g
Cinnamomi Cortex	4.0 g
Zizyphi Fructus	4.0 g
Glycyrrhizae Radix	2.0 g
Rhei Rhizoma	2.0 g
Zingiberis Rhizoma	1.0 g

• Usage=SHO

Used for those who have a relatively weak constitution with a distended abdomen, abdominal pain and constipation or diarrhea accompanied with tenesmus.

1) Although they pass stools there is a feeling of incomplete defecation.
2) Incomplete defecation after abdominal surgery.

COLOR PLATES

Treasures of the Tsumura Collection

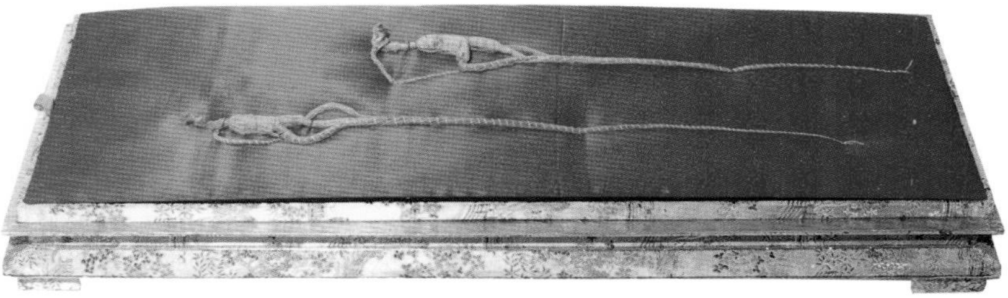

Ginseng known throughout the world as "The king of tonics"

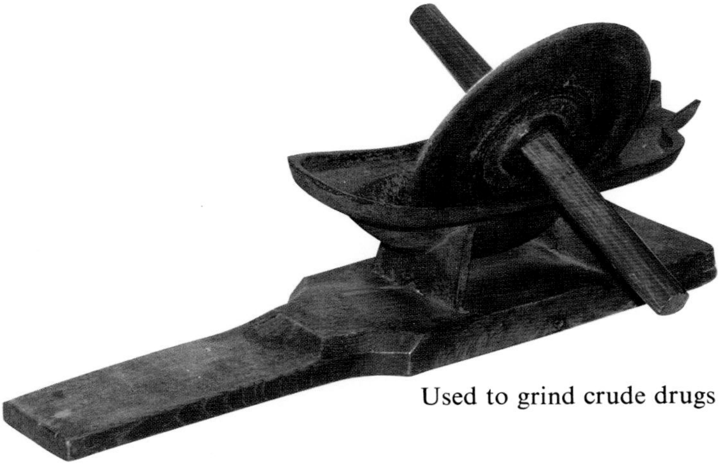

Used to grind crude drugs

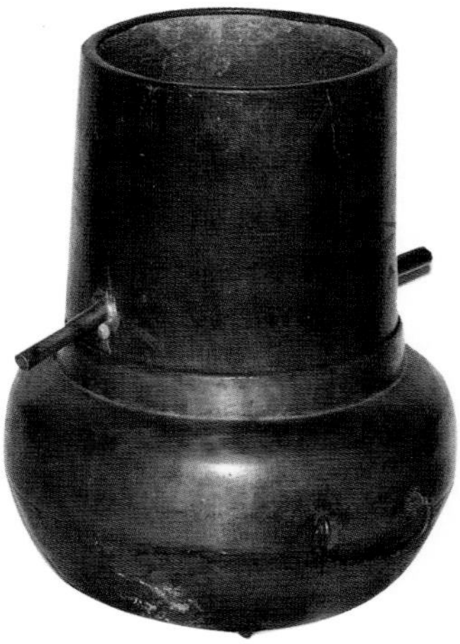

Kampo brewer mede of metal

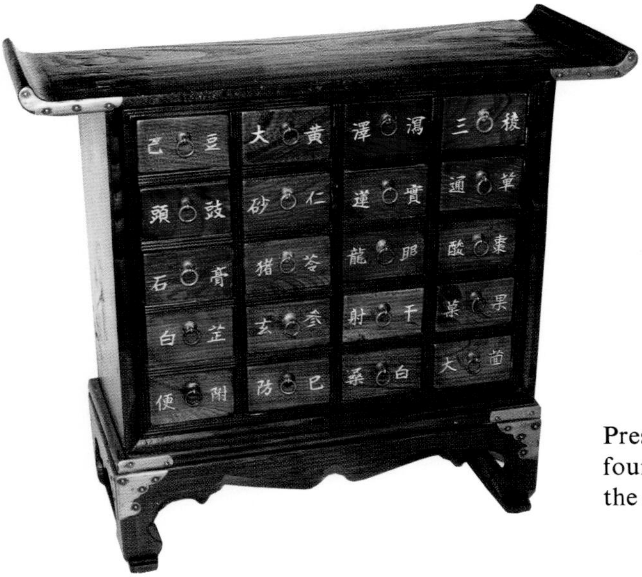

Prescription drawer chest found in pharmacies during the edo period

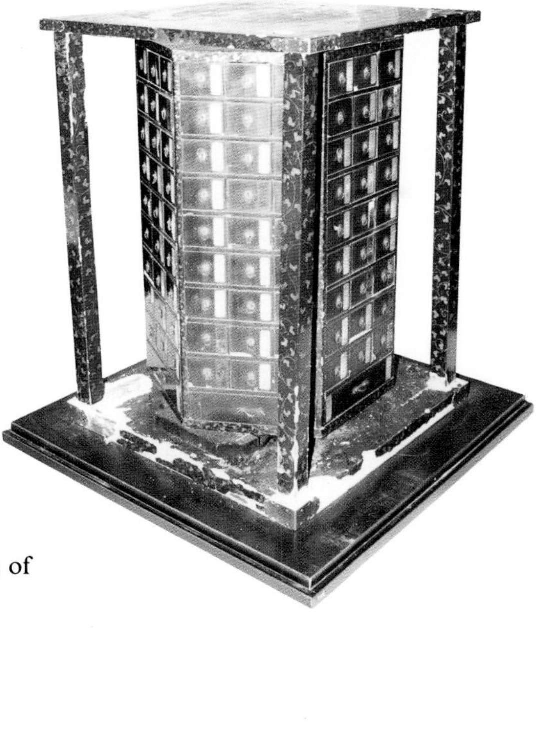

Revolving kampo drawers of this type are very rare

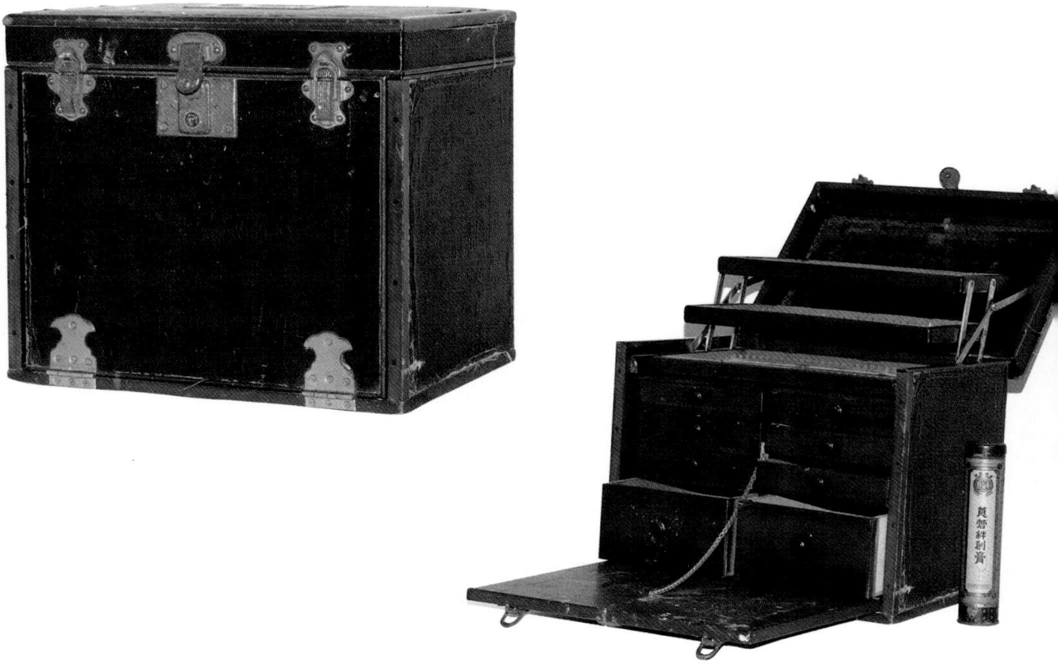

Medicine chests used once long ago

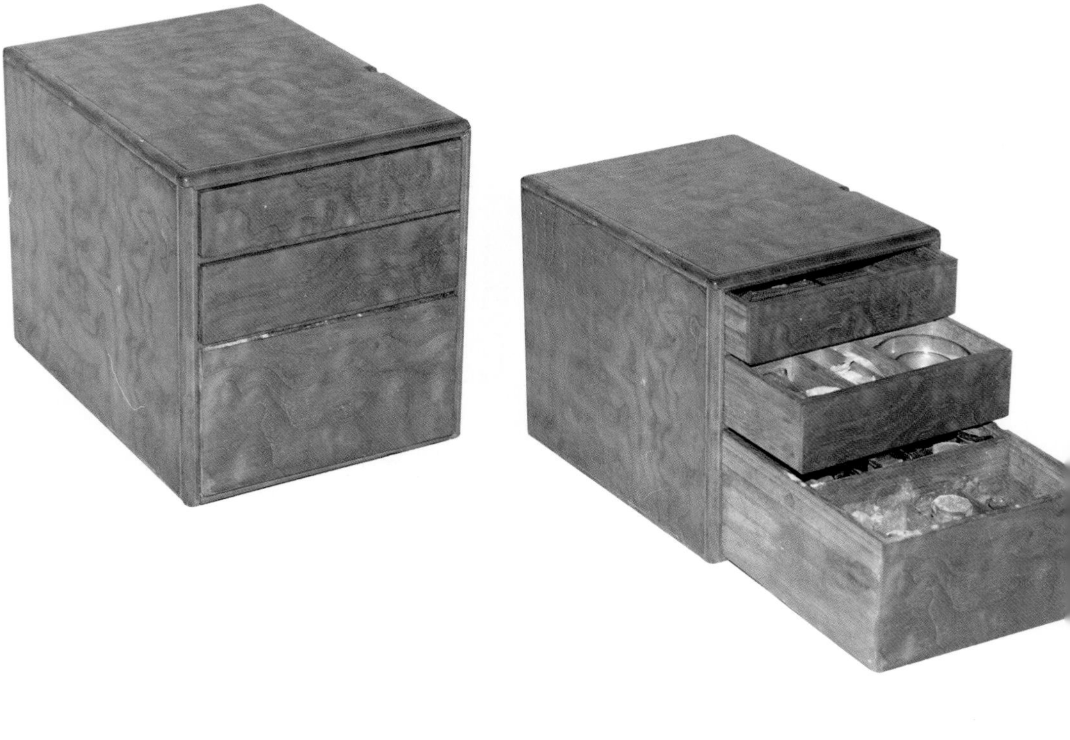

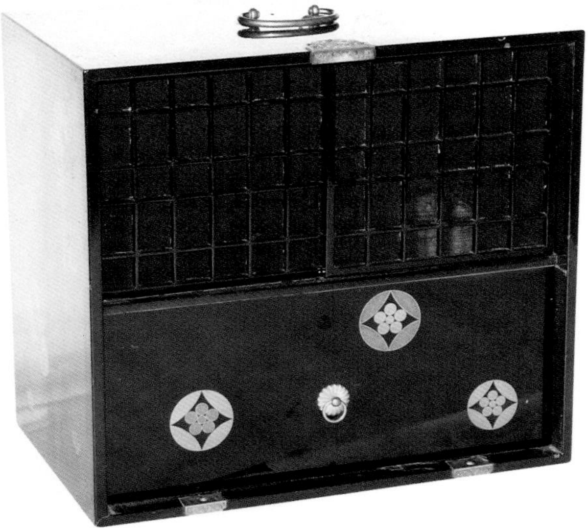

Portable 3 piece set containing
brewer and drawers for kampo

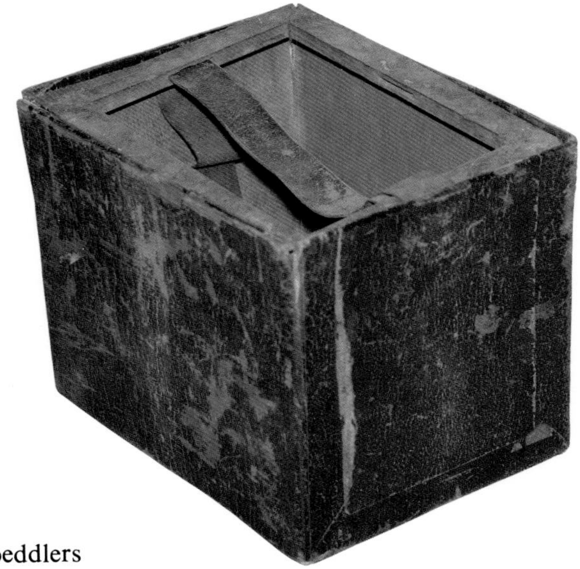

Medicine chest carried
on shoulders by kampo peddlers

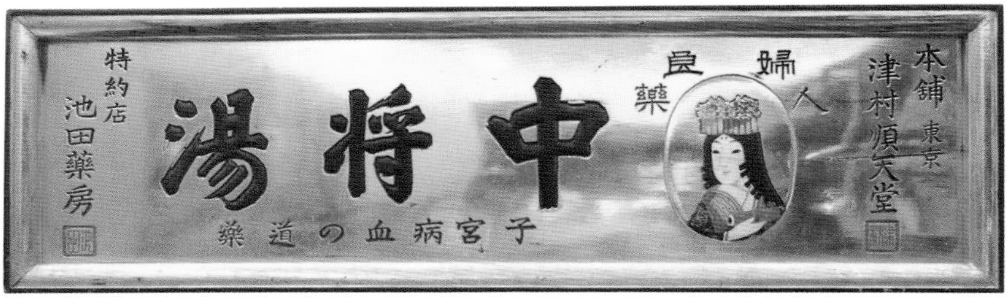

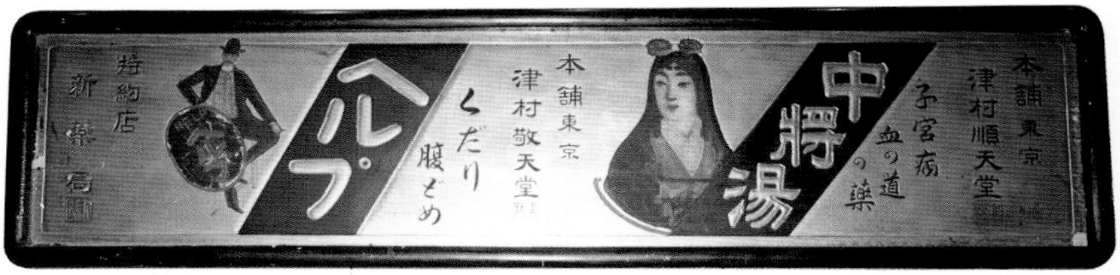

The Tsumura brand known throughout the country

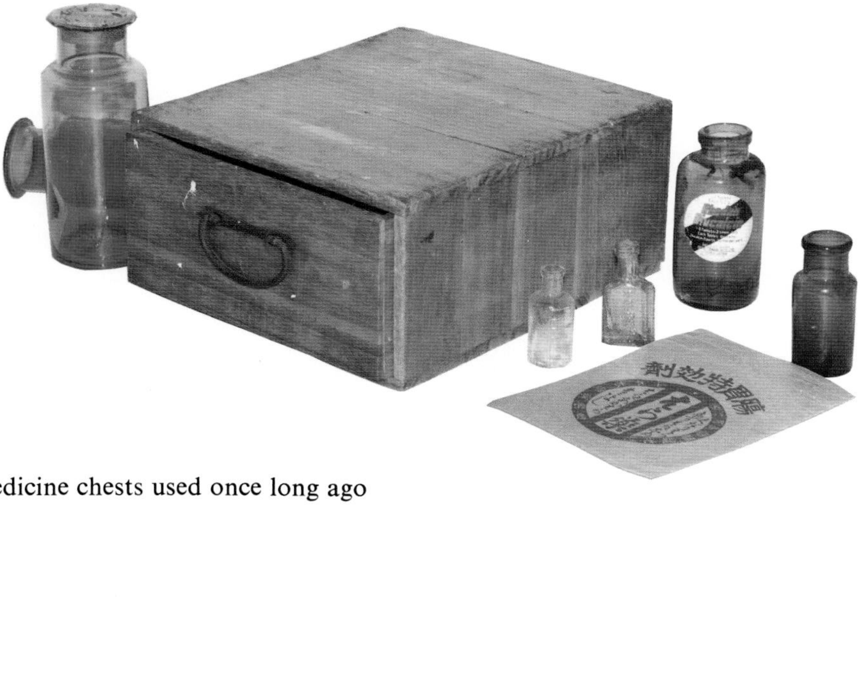

Medicine chests used once long ago

COLOR PLATES

Unrefined Drugs

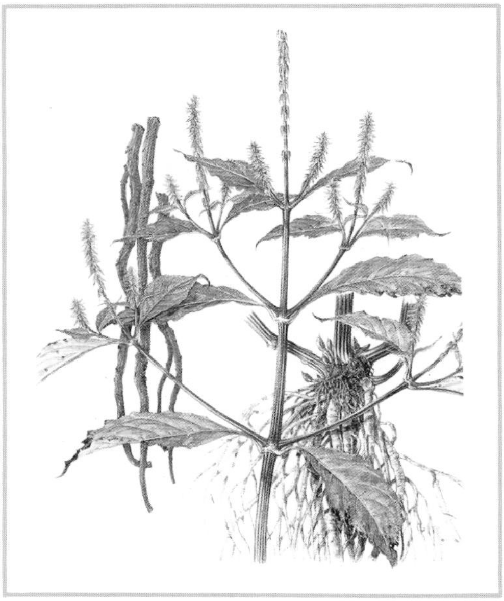

◀ **Achyranthis Radix**
[Origin] the root of *Achyranthes fauriei* LEV. et VAN'T or *A. bidentata* BL. of the Amaranthaceae family

Aconiti Tuber ▶
[Origin] the tuber of *Aconitum carmichaeli* DEBX. or other members of the Ranunculaceae family

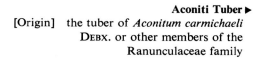

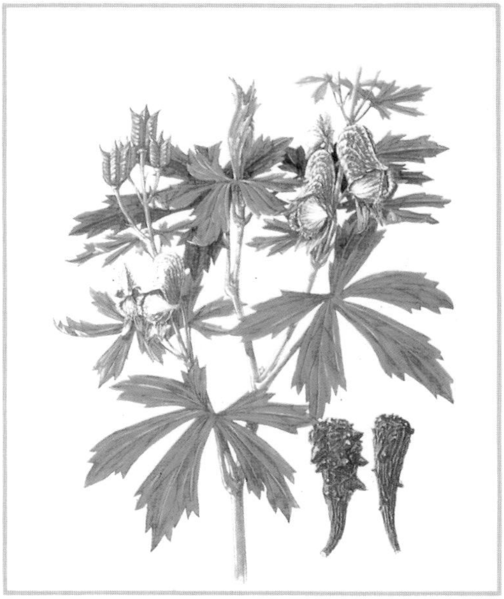

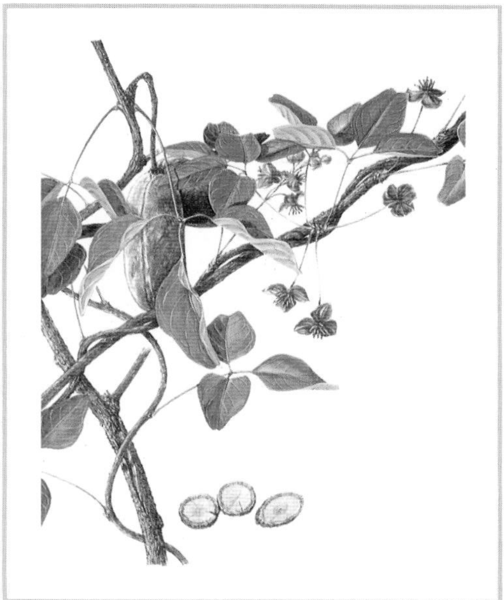

◀ **Akebiae Caulis**
[Origin] generally, the round sliced volubile stem of *Akebia quinata* DECANE. or other members of the Lardizabalaceae family

Alismatis Rhizoma ▶
[Origin] the tuber minus most of the stems, leaves, and roots of *Alisma orientale* JUZEPC. or similar members of the Alismataceae family

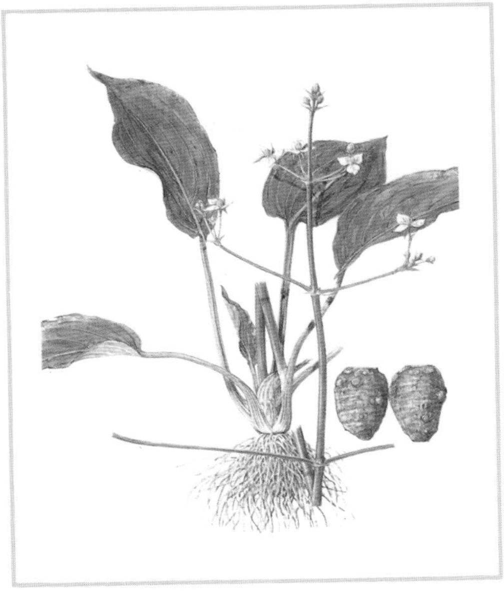

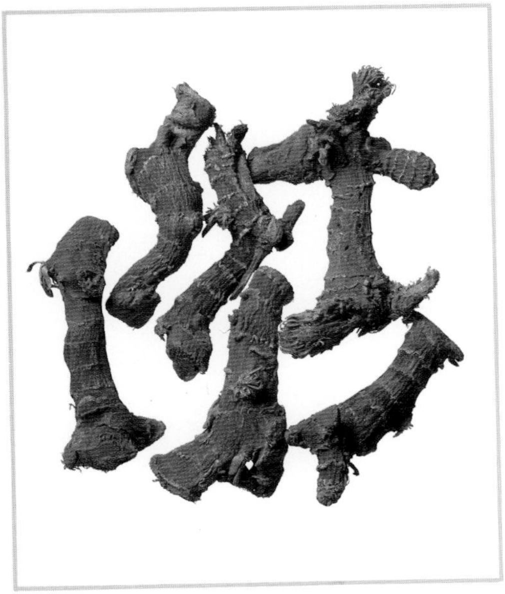

◀ Alpiniae Officinarum Rhizoma
[Origin] the rhizome of *Alpinia officinarum* HANCE of the Zingiberaceae family

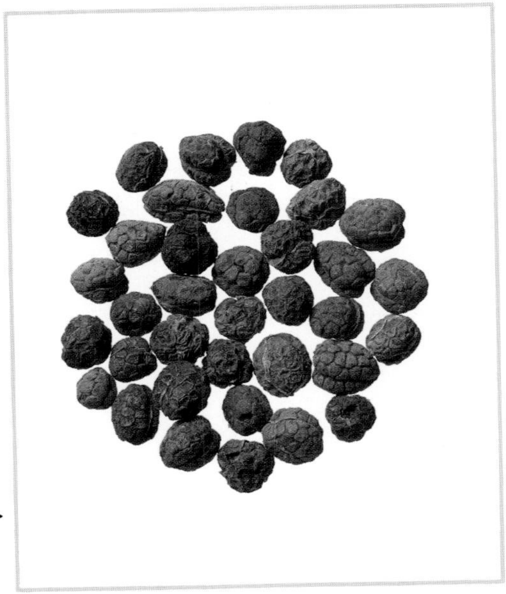

Amomi Semen ▶
[Origin] the seed of *Amomum xanthioides* WALL. of the Zingiberaceae family

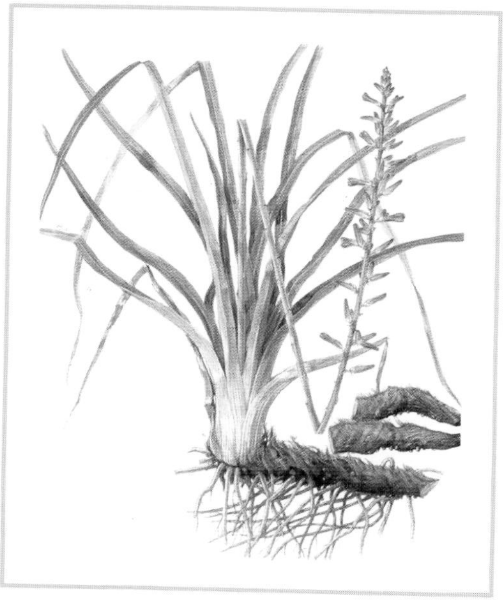

◀ **Anemarrhenae Rhizoma**
[Origin] the rhizome of *Anemarrhena asphodeloides* BGE. of the Liliaceae family

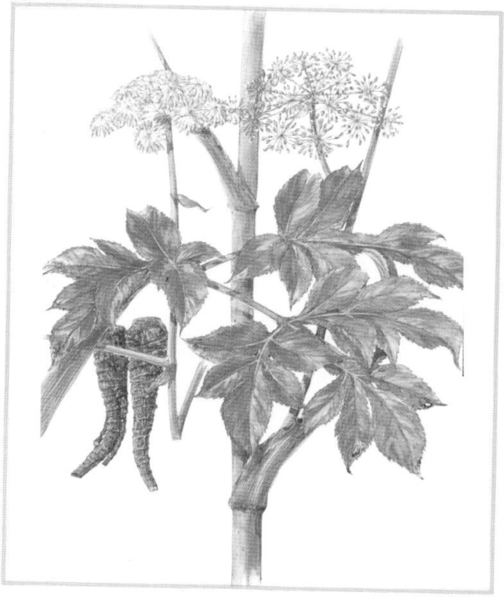

Angelicae Dahuricae Radix ▶
[Origin] the root of *Angelica dahurica* BENTH. et HOOK. or its varieties of the Umbelliferae family

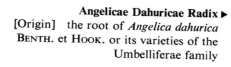

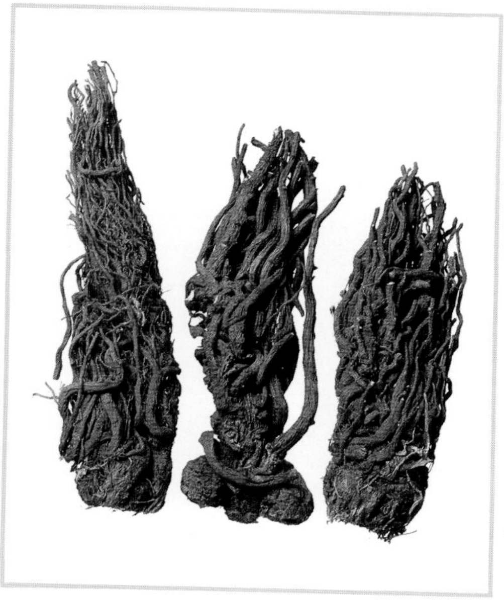

◀ **Angelicae Radix**
[Origin] generally, the steamed root of *Angelica acutiloba* KITAGAWA or similar members of the Umbelliferae family

Araliae Radix ▸
[Origin] the root *Aralia cordata* THUNB. of the Araliaceae family

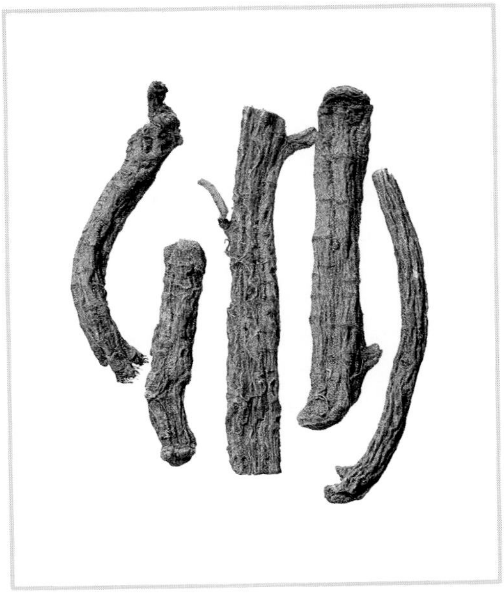

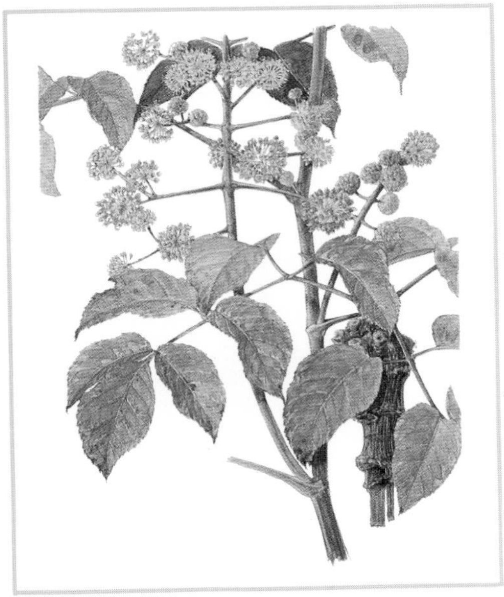

◂ Araliae Rhizoma et Radix
[Origin] generally, the rhizome of *Aralia cordata* THUNB. of the Araliaceae family

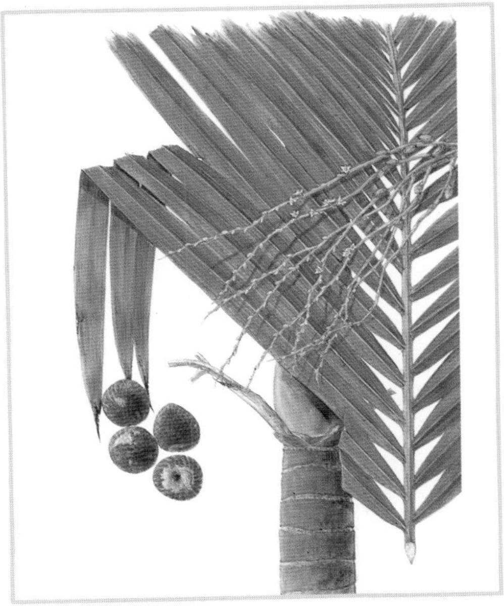

Arecae Semen ▸
[Origin] the seed of *Areca catechu* L. of the Palmae family

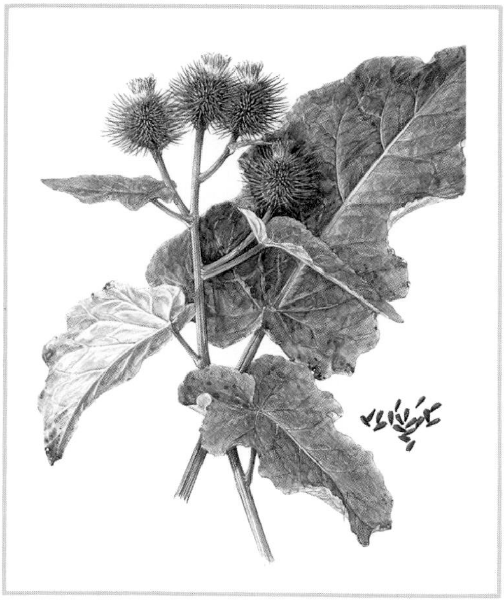

◀ **Arctii Fructus**
[Origin] the fruit of *Arctium lappa* L. of the Compositae family

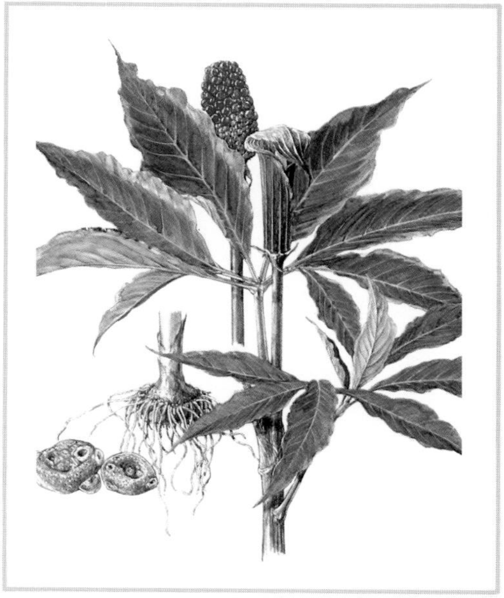

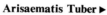

Arisaematis Tuber ▶
[Origin] the tuber minus the outer phelloderm of Arisaema japonicum BL., A. heterophyllum BL., or other members of the Araceae family

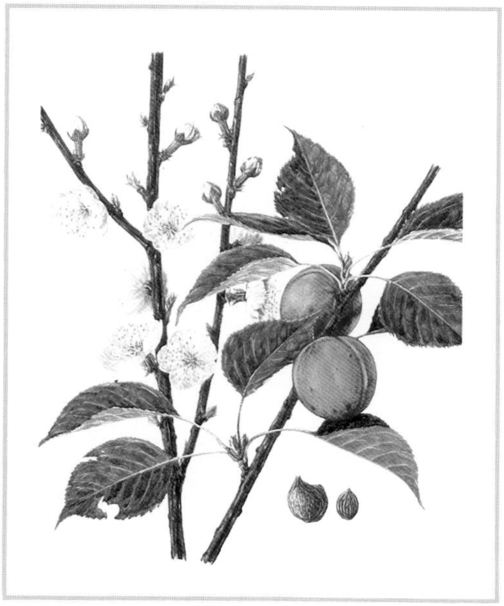

◀ **Armeniacae Semen**
[Origin] the seed of *Prunus armeniaca* L., *P. armeniaca* L. var. *ansu* MAXIM. or other similar members of the Rosaceae family

Artemisiae Folium ▸
[Origin] the leaf and the tip of the branch of *Artemisia princeps* PAMP. or *A. montana* PAMP. of the Compositae family

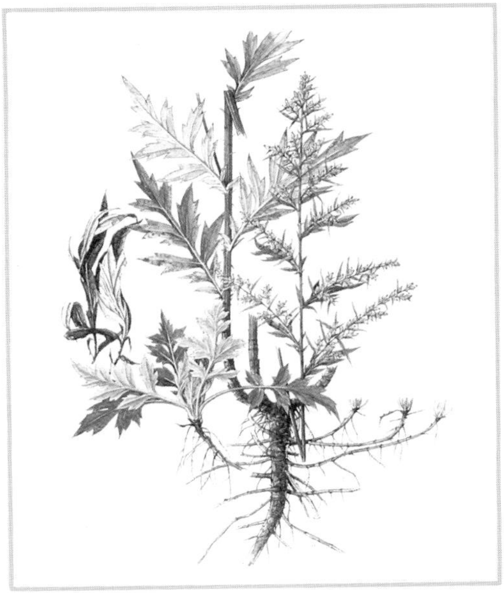

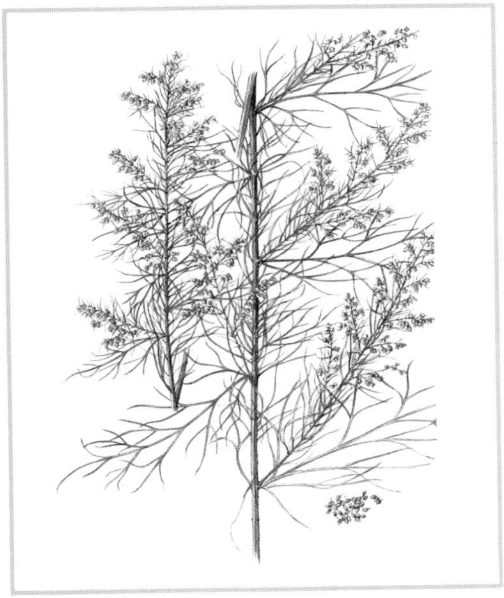

◂ Artemisiae Capillaris Spica
[Origin] the head of the flower of *Artemisia capillaris* THUNB. of the Compositae family

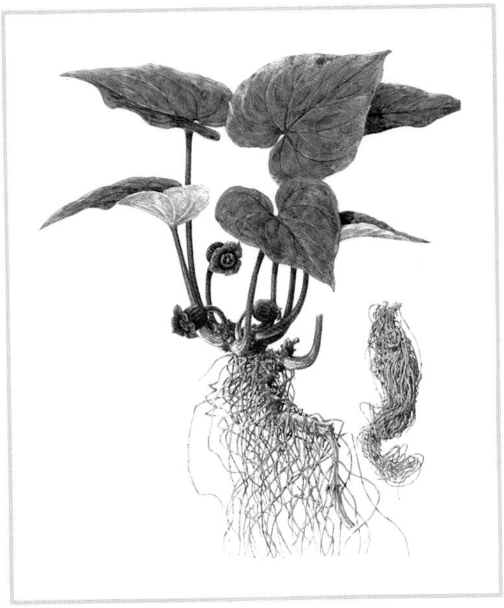

Asiasari Radix ▸
[Origin] the root and rhizome minus any part growing above-ground of *Asiasarum sieboldi* F. MAEKAWA or *Asiasarum heterotropoides* F. MAEKAWA var. *mandshuricum* F. MAEKAWA of the Aristolochiaceae family

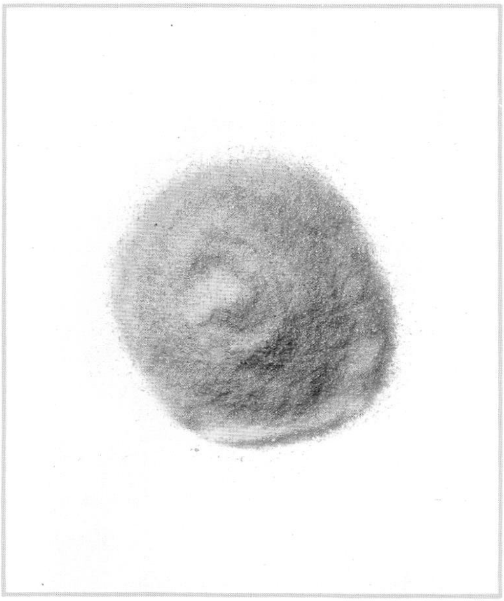

◀ **Asini Gelatinum**
[Origin] an extract of the hairless hide of *Equus aninus* L. or of the hide/bone/tendons/ligaments of other members of the Equidae family produced by heating, fat removal, concentration, and solidification

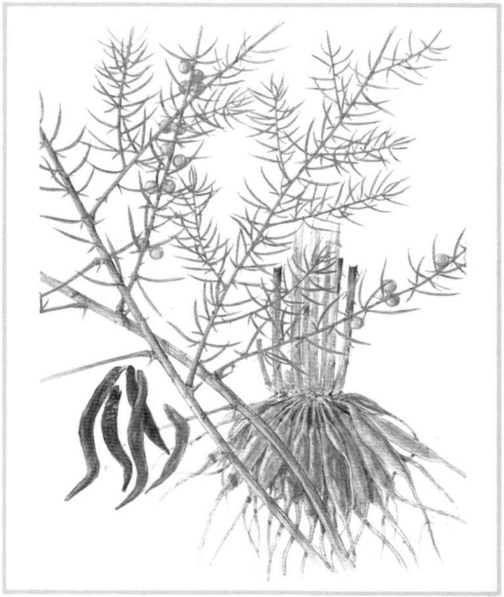

Asparagi Radix ▶
[Origin] the root minus the greater part of the outside phelloderm of *Aspargus* cochinchinensis Merr. of the Liliaceae family

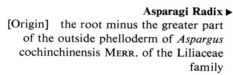

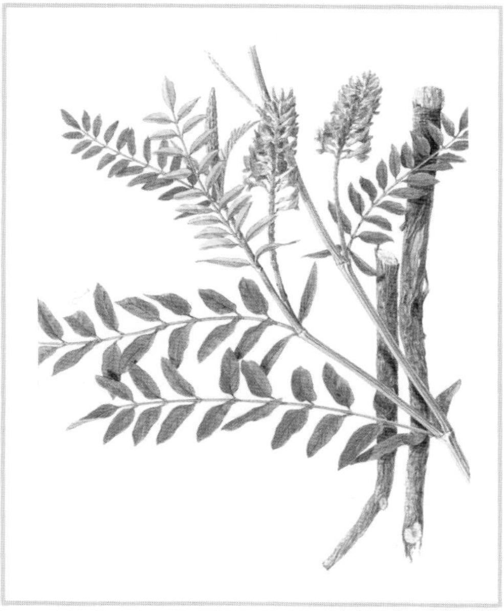

◀ **Astragali Radix**
[Origin] the root of *Astragalus membranaceus* Bge. or other members of the Leguminosae family

Atractylodis Lanceae Rhizoma ▶

[Origin] the rhizome of *Atractylodes lancea* DC. or its varieties, members of the Compositae family

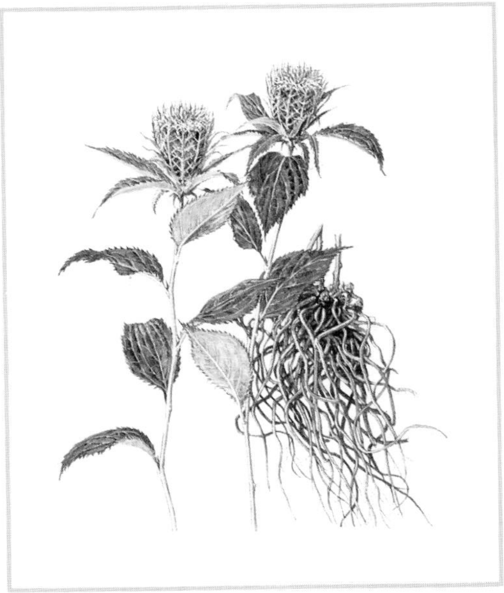

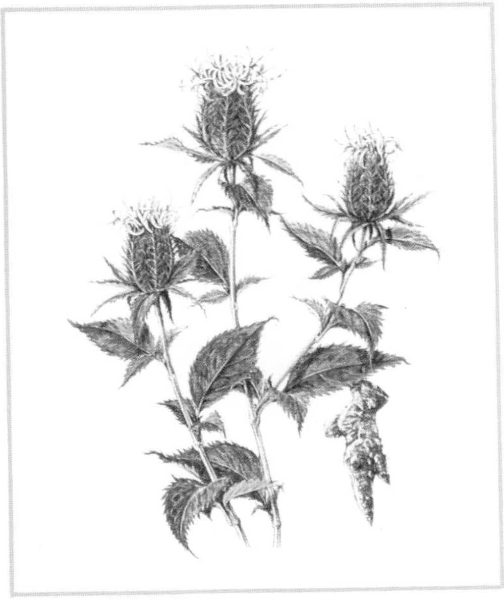

◀ Atractylodis Rhizoma

[Origin] generally, the Rhizome minus the pericerm of *Atractylodes japonica* KOIDZUMI or the rhizome or *A. ovata* DC. of the Compositae family

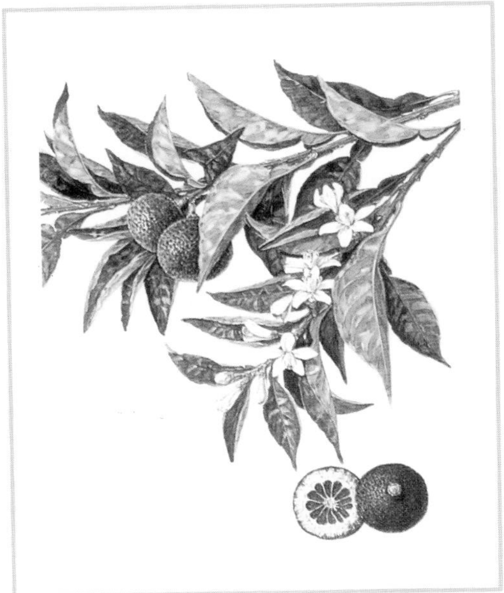

Aurantii Fructus Immaturus ▶

[Origin] the unripe fruit of *Citrus aurantium* L. var. *daidai* MAKINO, *C. natsudaidai* HAYATA, *C. unshiu* MARKOV, or other similar members of the Rutaceae family

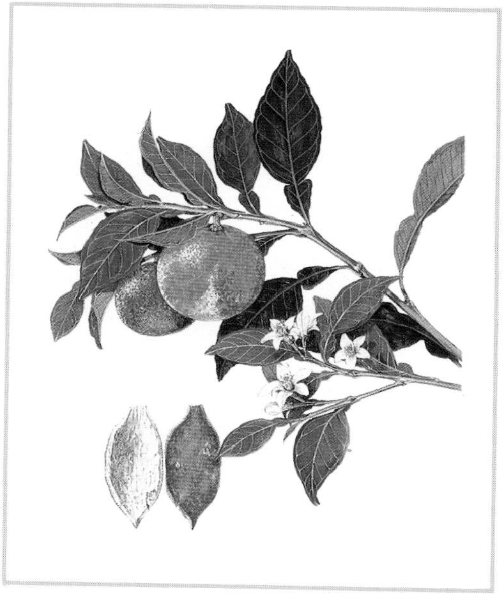

◀ **Aurantii Nobilis Pericarpium**
[Origin] the pericarp of the ripe fruit of *Citrus unshiu* MARKOV. or similar members of the Rutaceae family

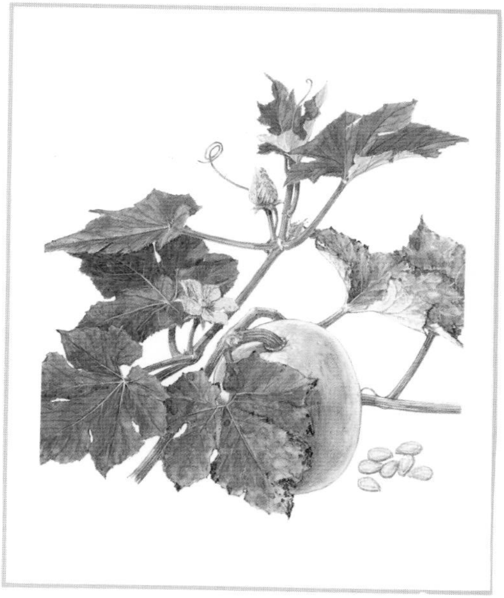

Benincasae Semen ▶
[Origin] the seed of *Benincasa cerifera* SAVI or *B. cerifera* SAVI. forma *emarginata* K. KIMURA et SUGIYAMA of the Cucurbitaceae family

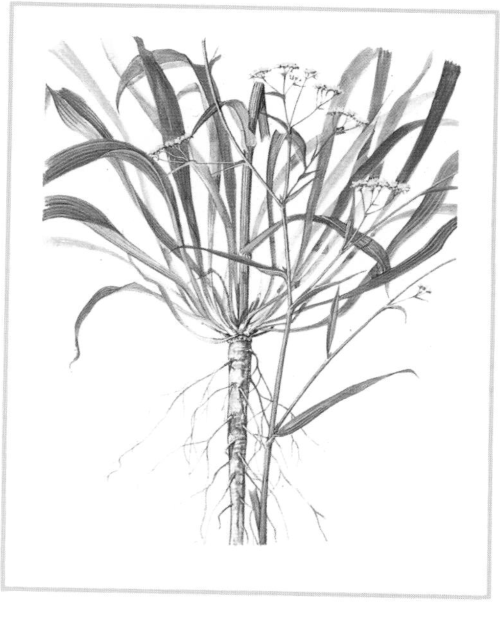

◀ **Bupleuri Radix**
[Origin] the root of ***Bupleurum falcatum*** L. or its varieties, members of the Umbelliferae family

Cannabidis Semen ▶
[Origin] the fruit of *Cannabis sativa* L. of the Moraceae family

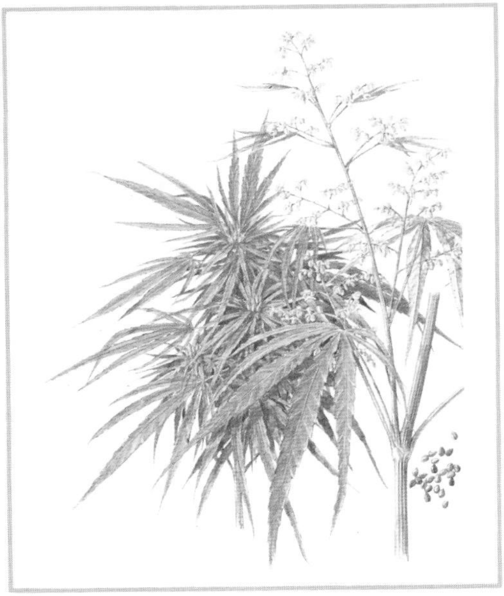

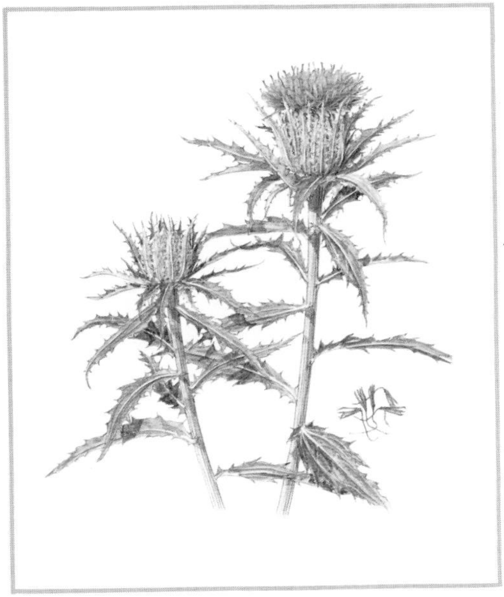

◀ Carthami Flos
[Origin] the tubulous blooming flower of *Carthamus tinctoritus* L. of the Compositae family

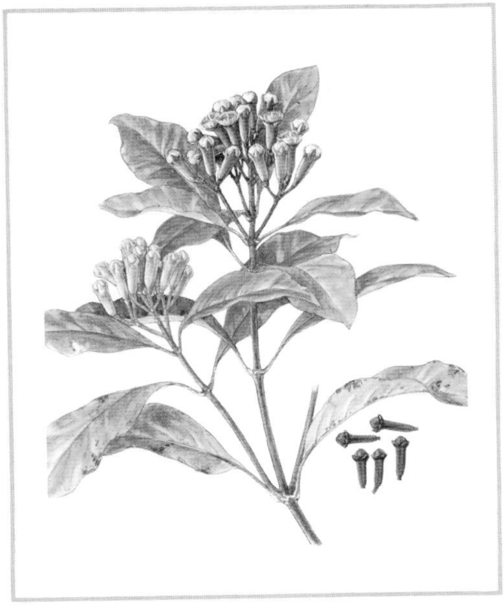

Caryophylli Flos ▶
[Origin] the bud of *Syzygium aromaticum* MERR. et PERRY. of the Myrtaceae family

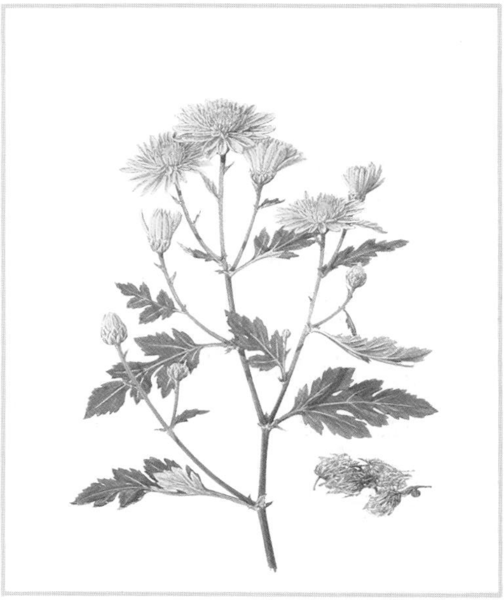

◀ **Chrysanthemi Flos**
[Origin] the head flowers of *Chrysanthemum indicum* L., *C. morifolium* RAMAT. or the crosses between these species of the Compositae family

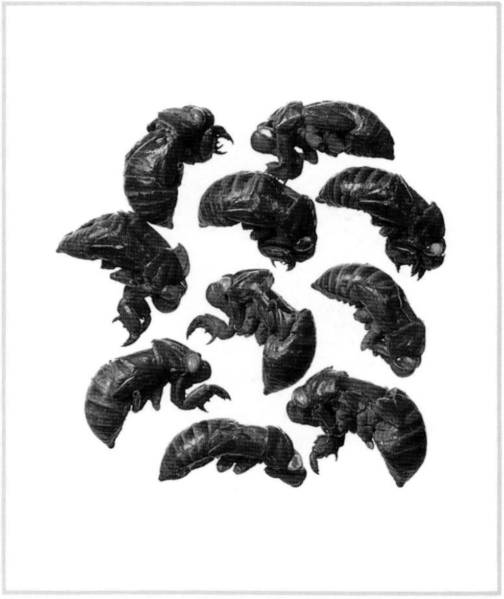

Cicadae Periostracum ▶
[Origin] the abandoned skin of the larva of *Cryptotympana pustulata* FABR. or other members of Cicadidae

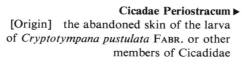

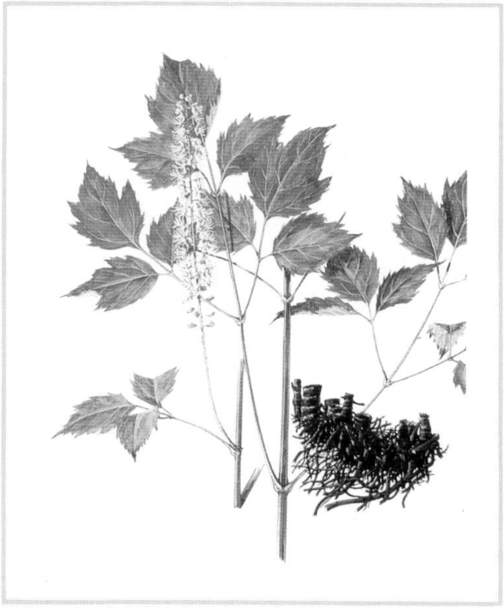

◀ **Cimicifugae Rhizoma**
[Origin] the rhizome of *Cimicifuga simplex* WORMSK. or other members of the Ranunculaceae family

Cinnamomi Cortex ▶
[Origin] the cortex of *Cinnamomum cassia* BL. or other plants of the Lauraceae family

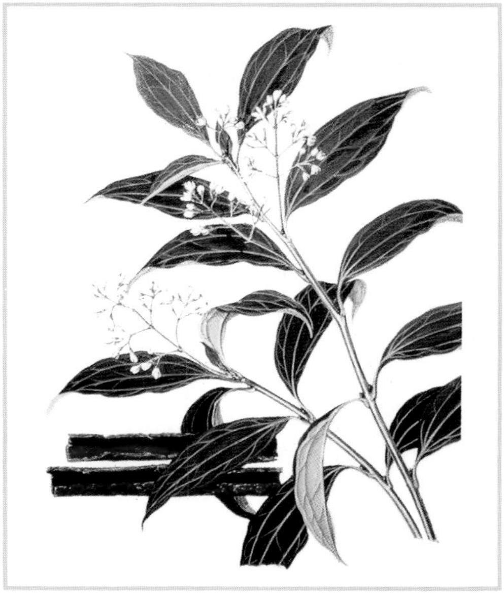

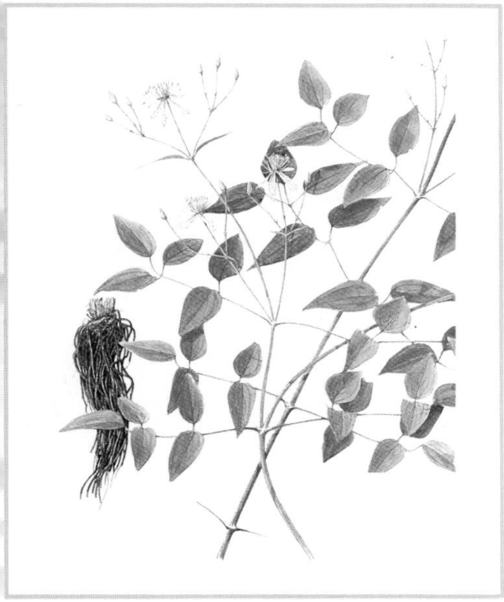

◀ Clematidis Radix
[Origin] the root and rhizome of *Clematis chinensis* OSBECK or similar members of the Ranunculaceae family

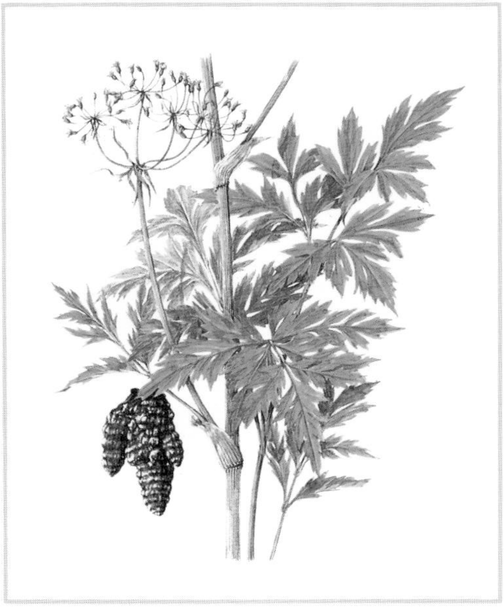

Cnidii Rhizoma ▶
[Origin] generally, the steamed rhizome of *Cnidium officinale* MAKINO of the Umbelliferae family

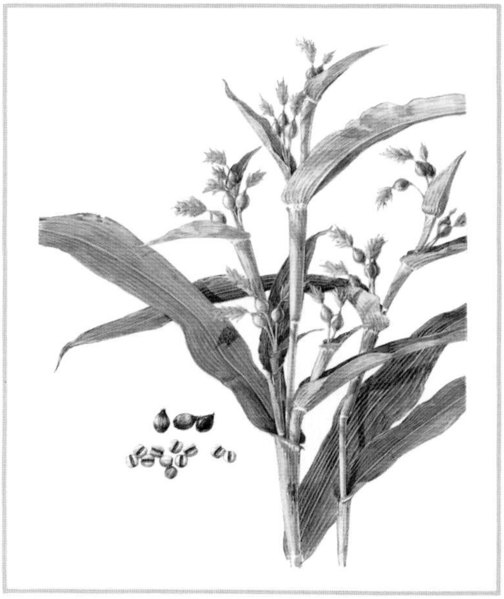

◀ **Coicis Semen**
[Origin] the seed minus its coat of *Coix lachryma-jobi* L. var. *ma-yuen* STAPF of the Gramineae family

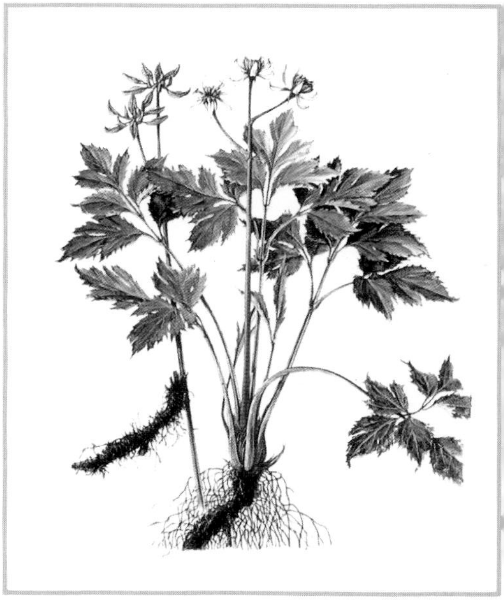

Coptidis Rhizoma ▶
[Origin] the rhizome minus most of the root of *Coptis japonica* MAKINO or other members of the Ranunculaceae family

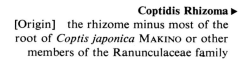

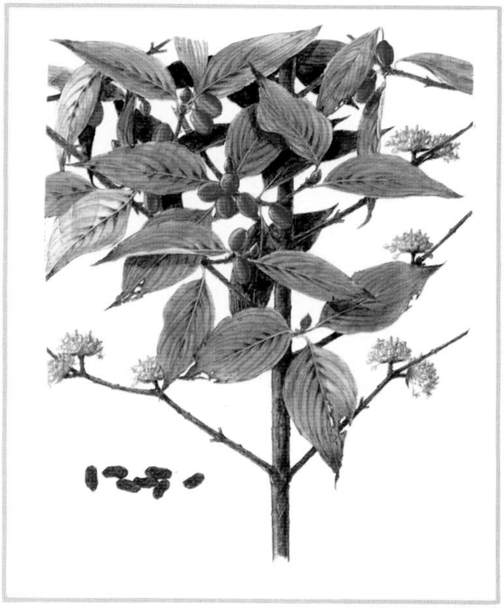

◀ **Corni Fructus**
[Origin] the flesh of the fruit minus most seeds of *Cornus officinalis* SIEB. et ZUCC. of the Cornaceae family

Corydalis Tuber ▸
[Origin] the rhizome of *Corydalis turtschaninouii* Bess. f. yanhusuo Y. H. chan et C. C. Hsu or other members of the Papaveraceae family

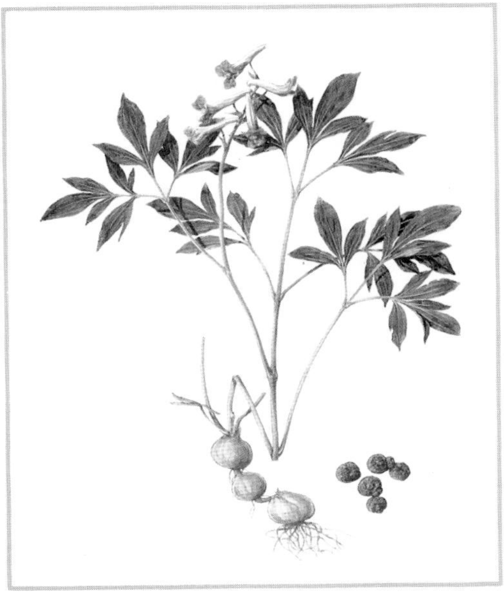

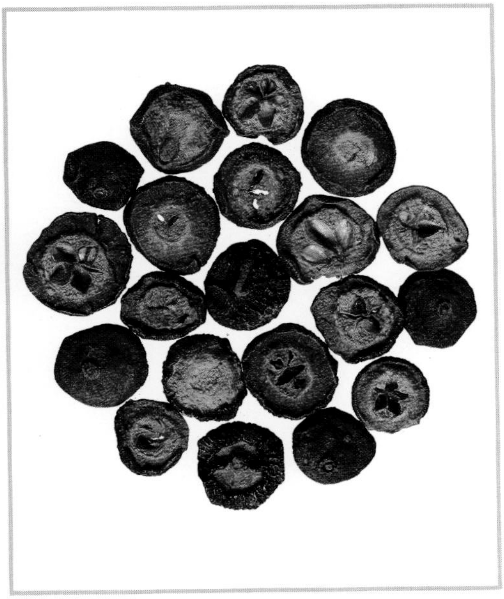

◂ Crataegi Fructus
[Origin] the fruit of *Crataegus cuneata* SIEB. et ZUCC. or other members of the Rosaceae family

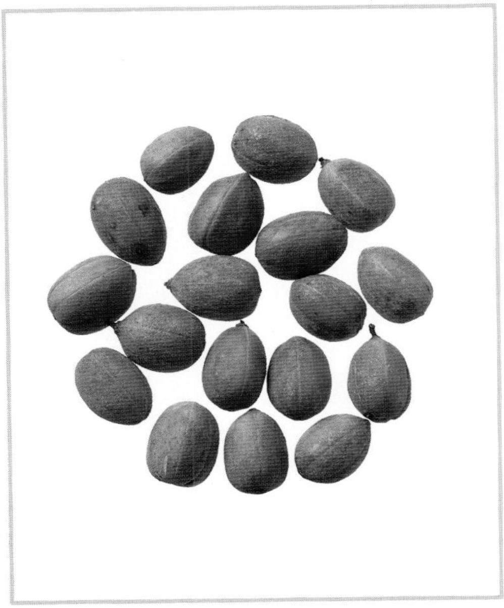

Crotonis Semen ▸
[Origin] the seed of *Croton tiglium* L. of the Euphorbiaceae family

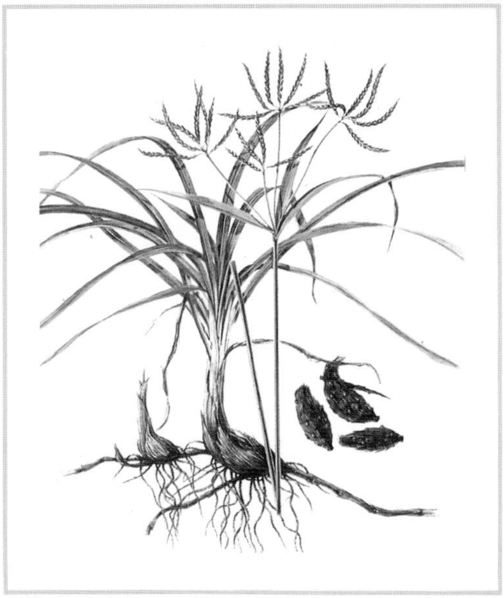

◀ **Cyperi Rhizoma**
[Origin] the rhizome minus the rootlets etc. of *Cyperus rotundus* L. of the Cyperaceae family

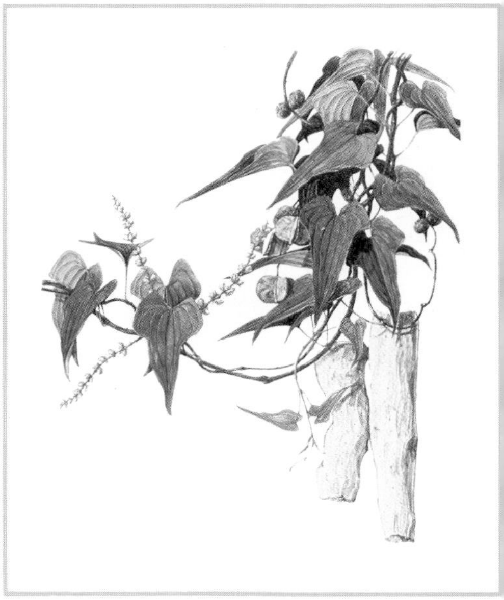

Dioscoreae Rhizoma ▶
[Origin] the rhizome (the root base) minus the periderm of *Dioscorea japonica* THUNB. or *Dioscorea batatas* DECNE of the Dioscoreaceae family

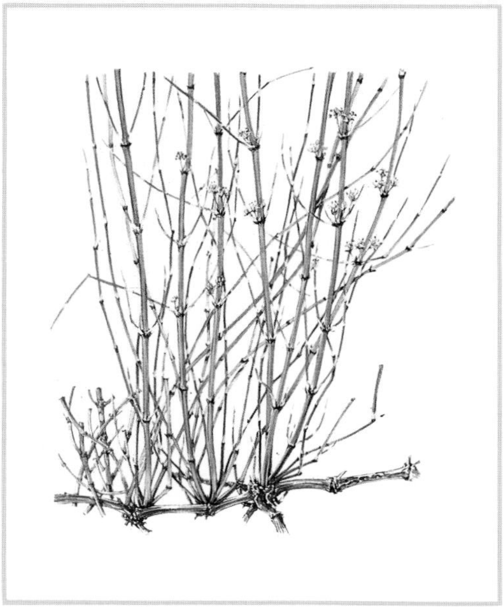

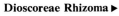

◀ **Ephedrae Herba**
[Origin] the stem of *Ephedra sinica* STAPF or other members of the Ephedraceae family

Eriobotryae Folium ▸
[Origin] the leaf of *Eriobotrya japonica* Lindl. of the Rosaceae family

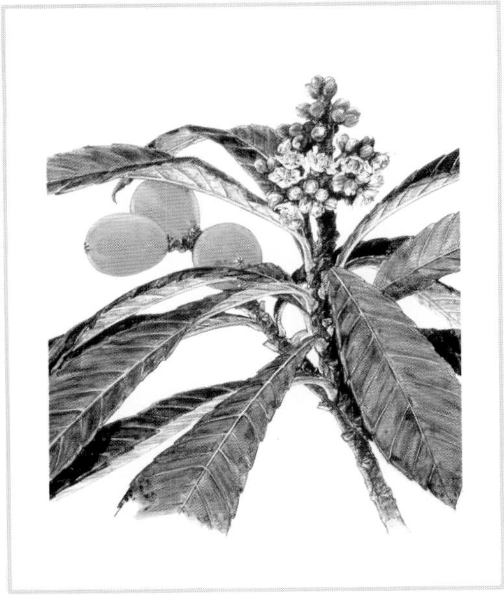

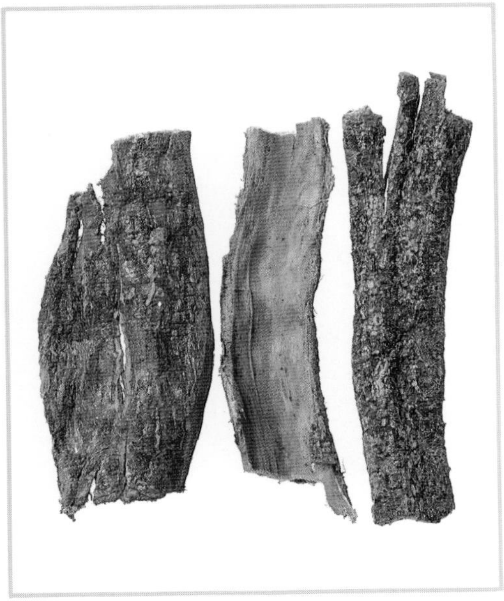

◂ Eucommiae Cortex
[Origin] the cortex of *Eucommia ulmoides* Oliv. of the Eucommiaceae family

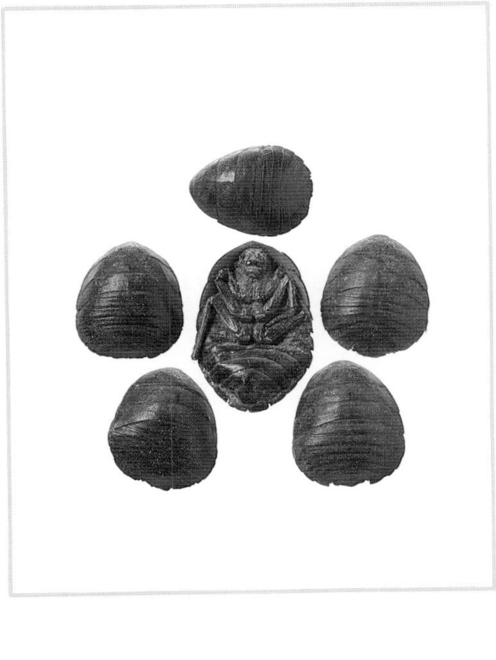

Eupolyphaga ▸
[Origin] the female *Eupolyphaga sinensis* Walker or *Opisthoplatia orientalis* Burm. of the Blattidae family

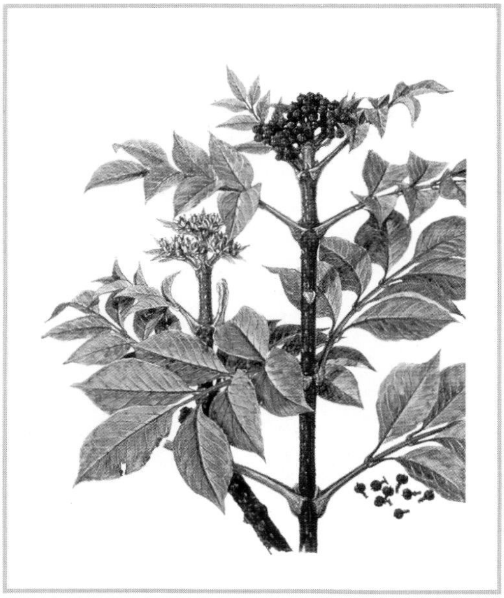

◀ **Evodiae Fructus**
[Origin] the fruit of *Evodia rutaecarpa* BENTH or *E. officinalis* DODE of the Rutaceae family

Fel Ursi ▶
[origin] the dried bile of *Ursus arctos* L. or similar members of the Ursidae family
(Note: The gallbladder is pictured.)

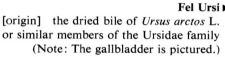

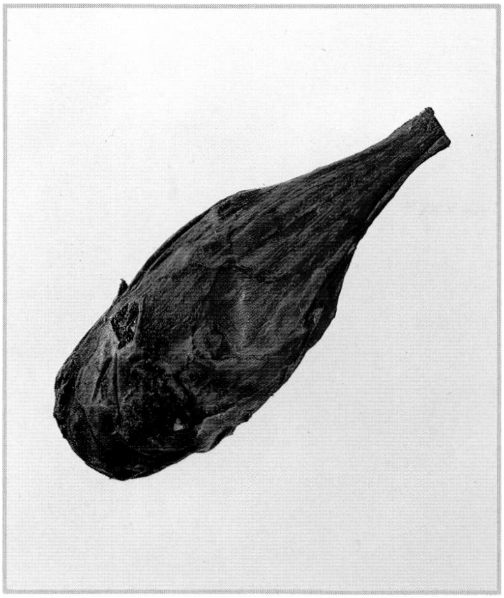

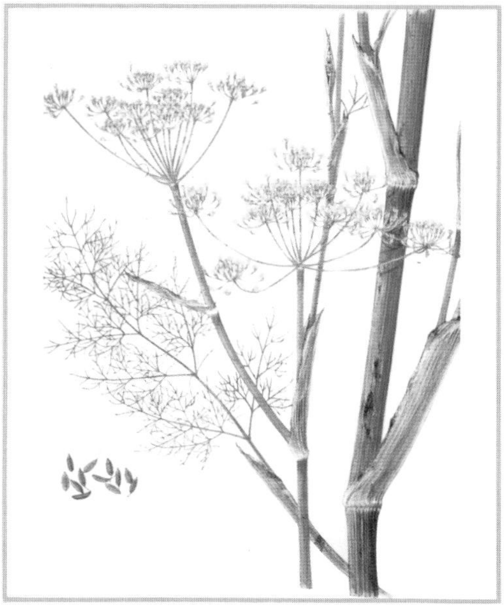

◀ **Foeniculi Fructus**
[Origin] the fruit of *Foeniculum vulgare* MILL. of the Umbelliferae family

Forsythiae Fructus ▶
[Origin] the fruit of *Forsythia suspensa* VAHL., *F. viridissima* LINDL. or *F. koreana* NAKAI of the Oleaceae family

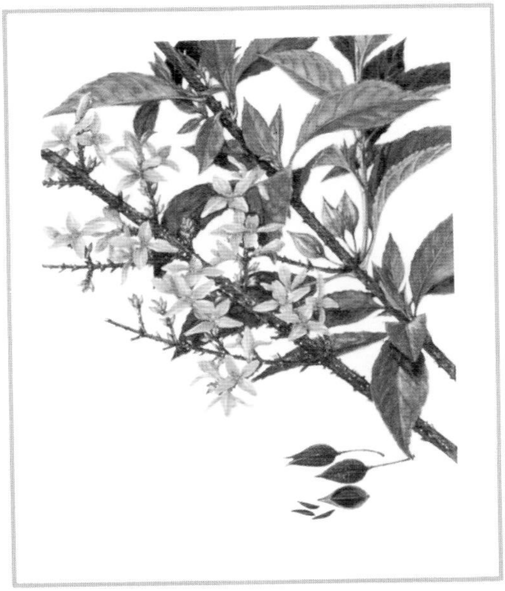

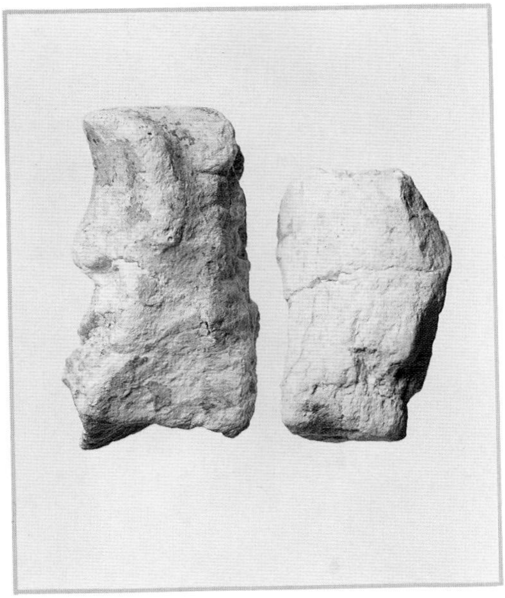

◀ Fossilia Ossis Mastodi
[Origin] the petrified bone of large mammals, mainly composed of calcium carbonate.

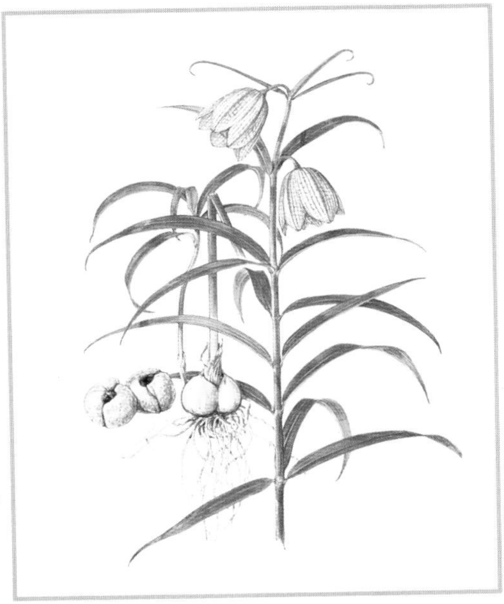

Fritillariae Bulbus ▶
[Origin] the bulb of *Fritillaria verticillata* WILLD. var. *thunbergii* BAK. of the Liliaceae family

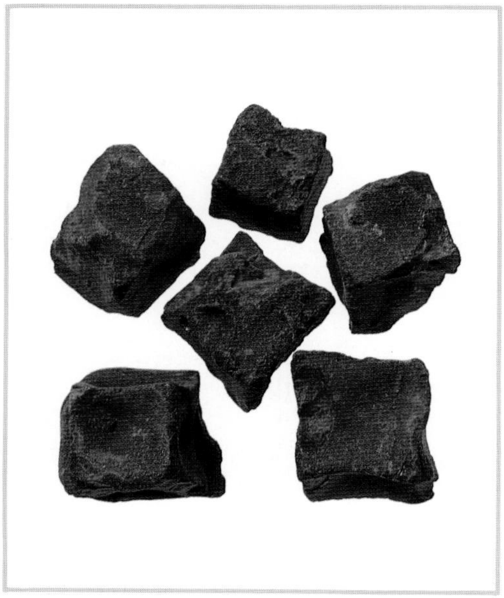

◀ **Gambir**
[Origin] a dried extract obtained from the leaves and young branches of *Uncaria gambir* ROXB. of the Rubiaceae family

Gardeniae Fructus ▶
[Origin] the fruit of *Gardenia jasminoides* ELLIS or other members of the Rubiaceae family

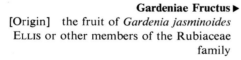

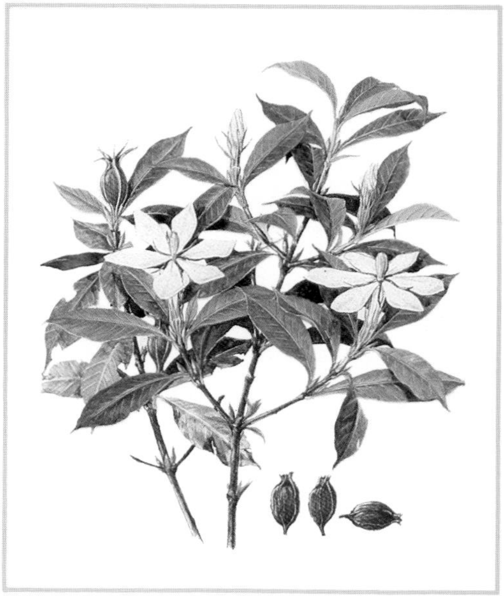

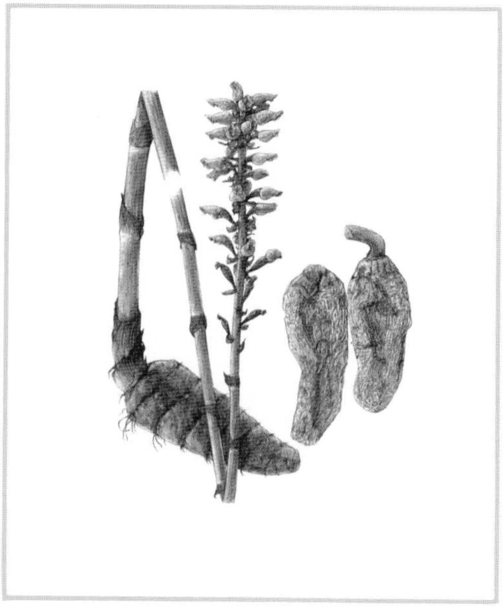

◀ **Gastrodiae Tuber**
[Origin] the tuber of *Gastrodia elata* BL. of the Orchidaceae family

Gentianae Scabrae Radix ▶
[Origin] the root and rhizome of *Gentiana scabra* BGE or other members of the Gentianaceae family

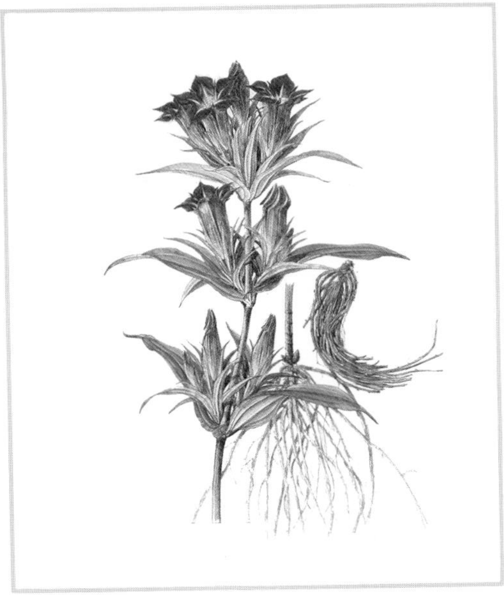

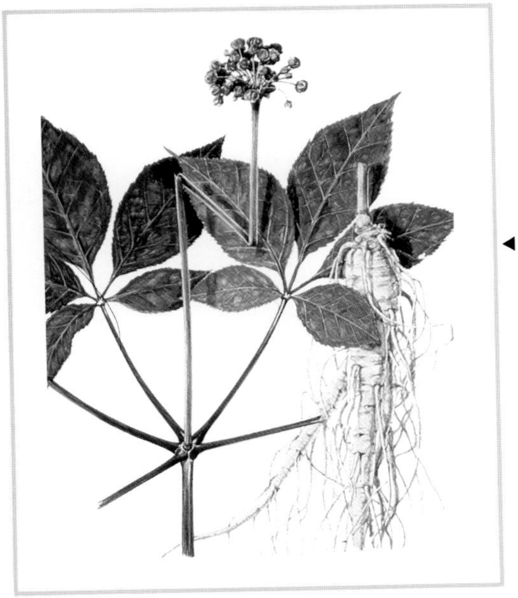

◀ Ginseng Radix
[Origin] the root minus the rootlets or the root steamed slightly of *Panax ginseng* C.A. MEY. of the Araliaceae family

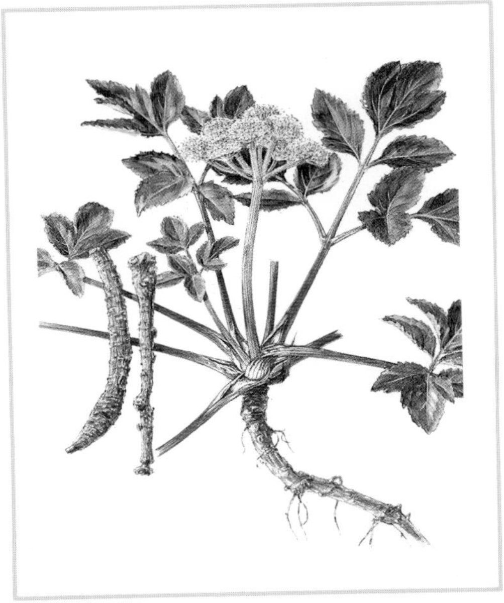

Glehniae Radix cum Rhizoma ▶
[Origin] the root and rhizome of *Glehnia littoralis* FR. SCHM-ex MIQ. of the Umbelliferae family

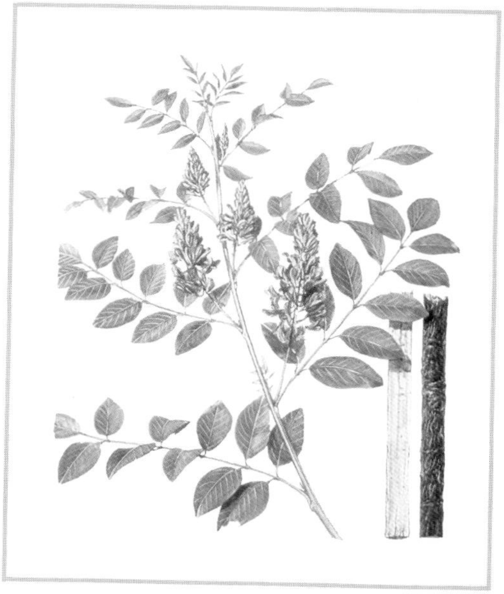

◀ **Glycyrrhizae Radix**
[Origin] the root and stolon of *Glycyrrhiza glabra* L. var. *glandulifera* REG. et HERD, or *G. uralensis* FISCH. or other members of the Leguminosae family

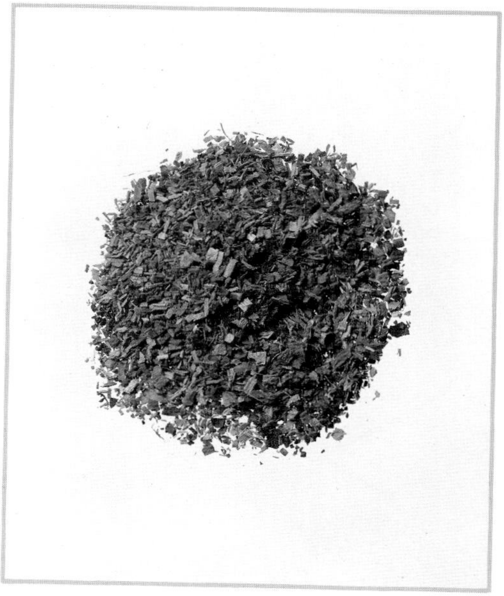

Glycyrrhizae Radix ▶
[Origin] the root and stolon of *Glycyrrhiza glabra* L. var. *glandulifera* REG. et HERD, *G. uralensis* FISCH. or other members of the Leguminosae family, warmed over a fire

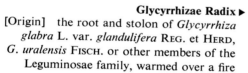

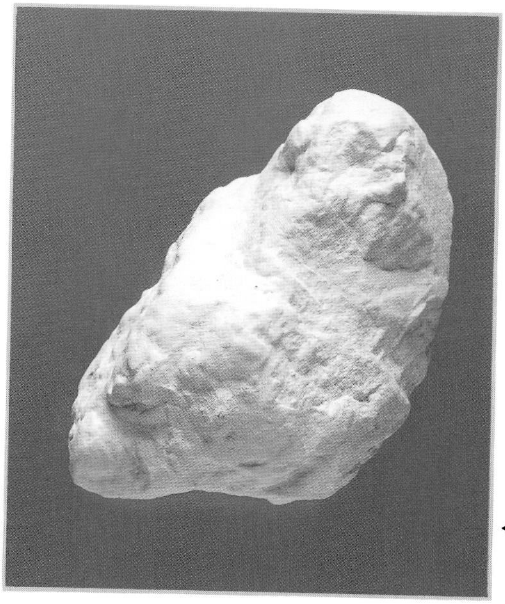

◀ **Gypsum Fibrosum**
[Origin] natural hydrous calcium sulfate, consisting almost entirely of $CaSO_4 \cdot 2H_2O$

Hoelen ▸
[Origin] generally, the sclerotium minus most of its outside layer of *Poria cocos* WOLF of the Polyporaceae family

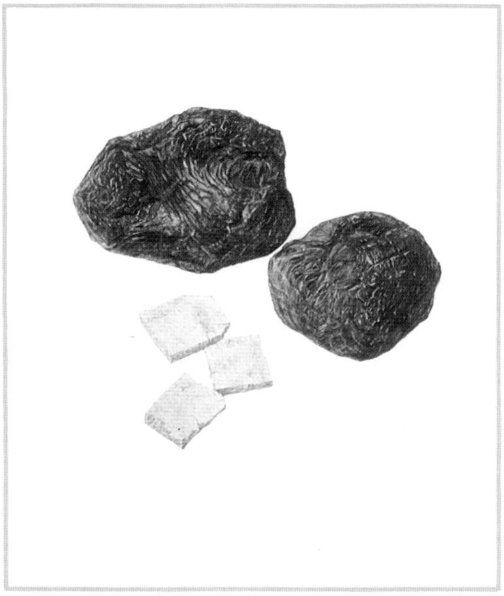

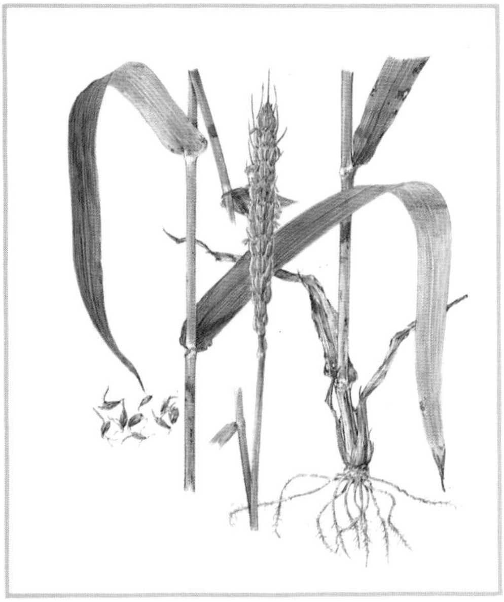

◂ Hordei Fructus Germinatus
[Origin] the seed of *Hordeum vulgare* L. var. *hexastion* ASCHERS. of the Gramineae family

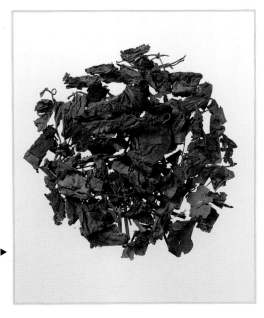

Houttuyniae Herba ▸
[Origin] the above-ground portion during the flowering season of *Houttuynia cordata* THUNB. of the Saururaceae family

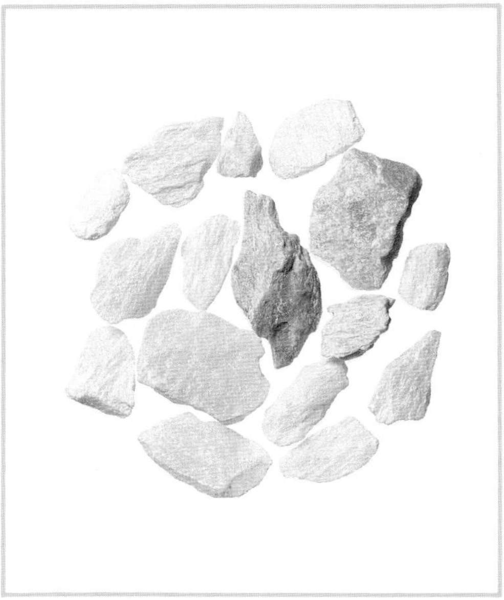

◀ **Kadinum**
[Origin] clayey minerals consisting mainly of hydrous aluminum silicate and silicon dioxide, or hydrohaloside
$Al_2O_3 \cdot 2SiO_2 \cdot 2H_2O \cdot 2H_2O$

Ledebouriellae Radix ▶
[Origin] the root and rhizime of *Ledebouriella seseloides* WOLF(F). of the Umbelliferae family

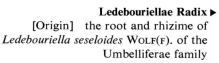

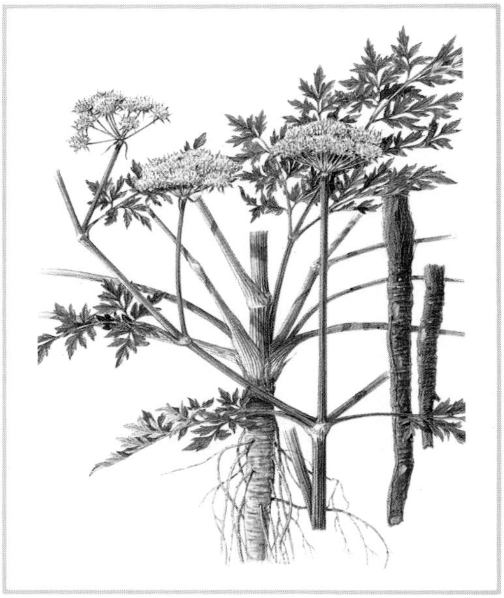

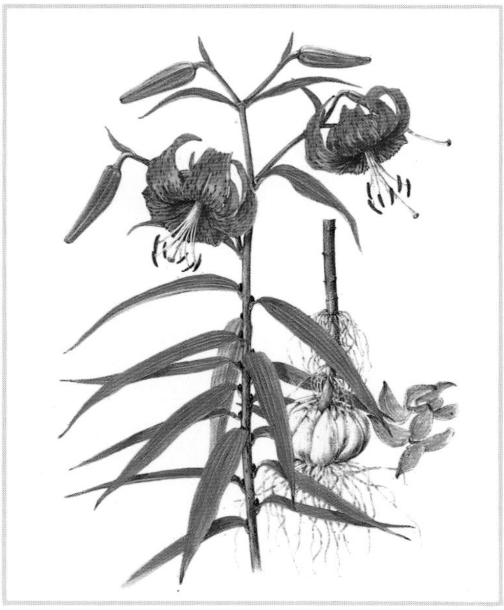

◀ **Lilii Bulbus**
[Origin] the rementum of *Lilium lancifolium* THUNB., *L. brownii* F. E. BROWN var. *colchesteri* WILS., or other members of the Liliaceae family

Lithospermi Radix ▶
[Origin] the root of *Lithospermum erythrorhizon* SIEB. et ZUCC. (hard) or *Macrotomia euchroma* PAULS (soft) of the Boraginaceae family

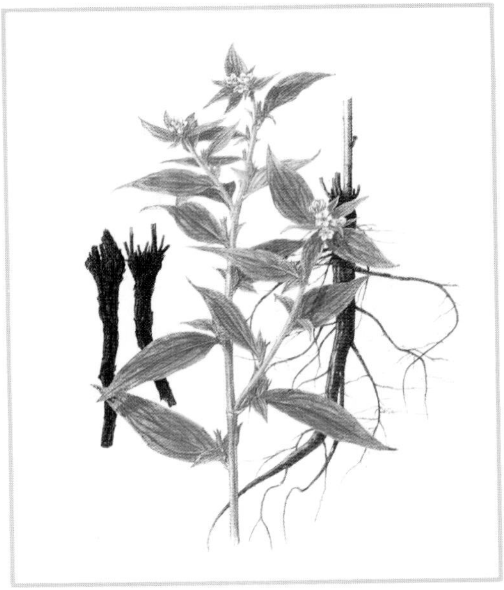

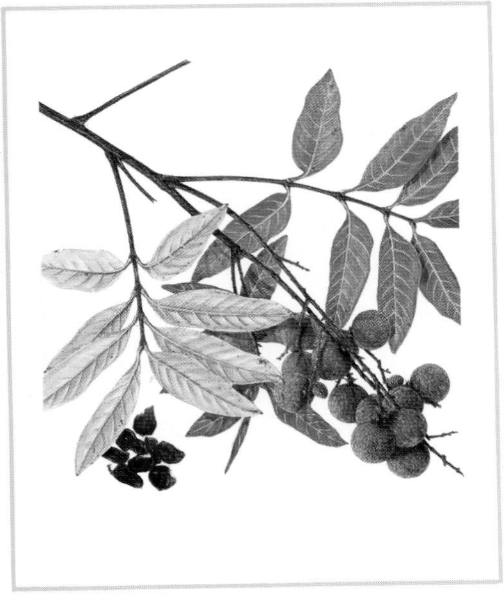

◀ Longanae Arillus
[Origin] the aril of *Euphoria longana* Lam. of the Sapindaceae family

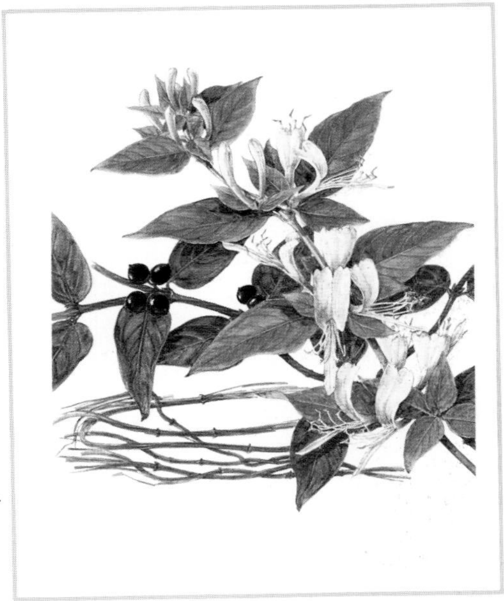

Lonicerae Caulis et Folium ▶
[Origin] the leaf and the stem of *Lonicera japonica* THUNB. of the Caprifoliaceae family

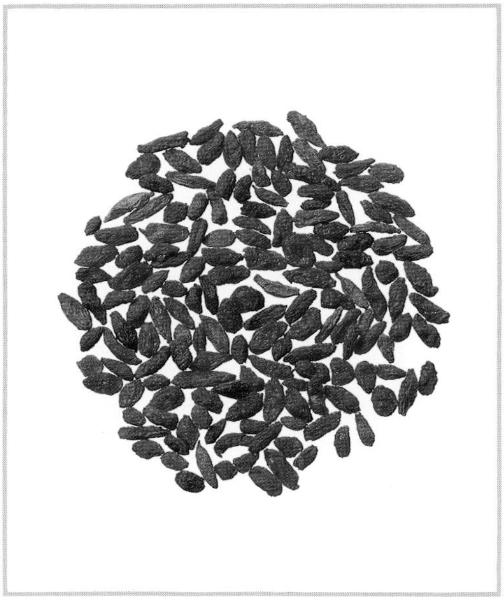

◀ **Lycii Fructus**
[Origin] the fruit of *Lycium chinense* MILL. of the Solanaceae family

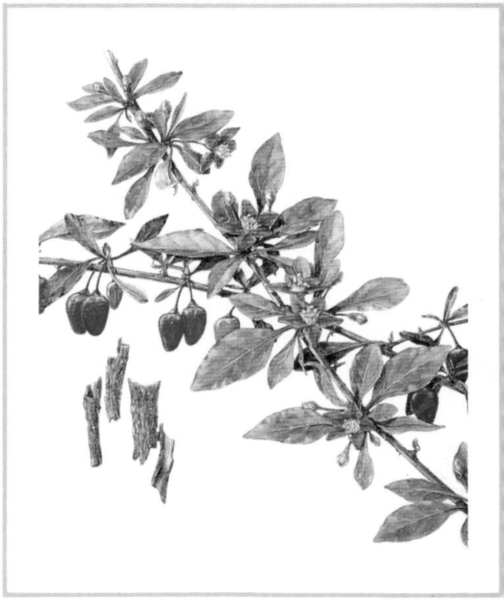

Lycii Radicis Cortex ▶
[Origin] the cortex of the root of *Lycium chinense* MILL. of the Solanaceae family

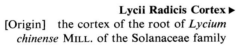

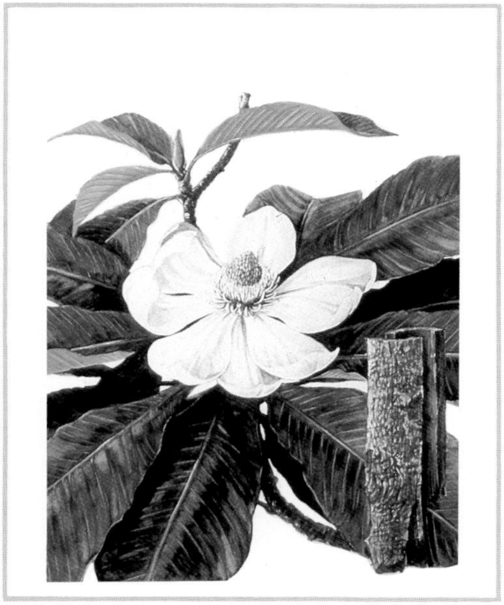

◀ **Magnoliae Cortex**
[Origin] the cortex of *Magnolia obovata* THUNB. of the Magnoliaceae family

Magnoliae Flos ▸
[Origin] the bud of *Magnolia saliciflora* MAXIM., M. kobus DC. or other similar members of the Magnoliaceae family

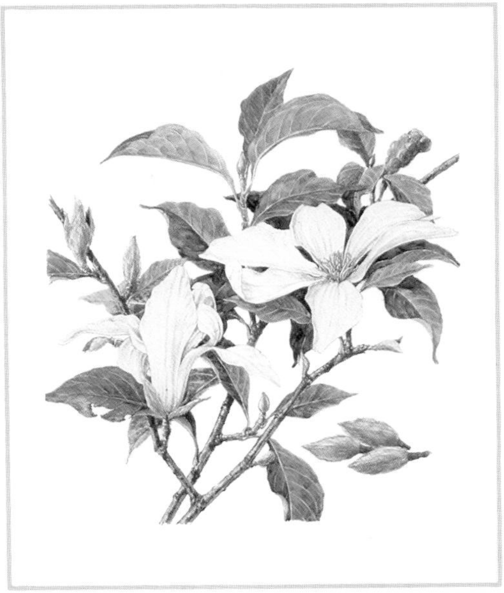

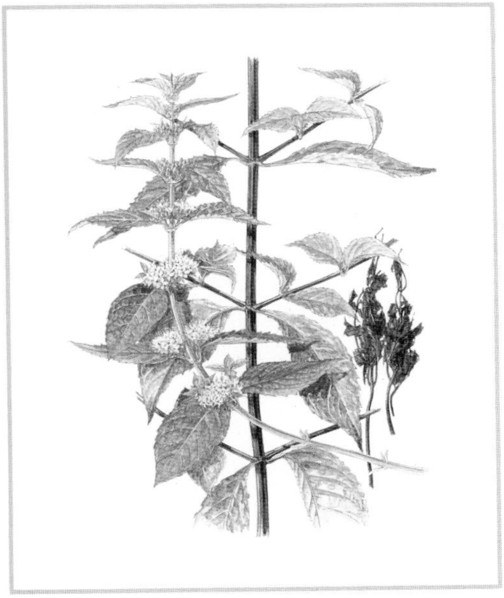

◂ Menthae Herba
[Origin] the part on the ground of *Mentha arvensis* L. var. *piperascens* MALINVAUD or the crosses between its species of the Labiatae family

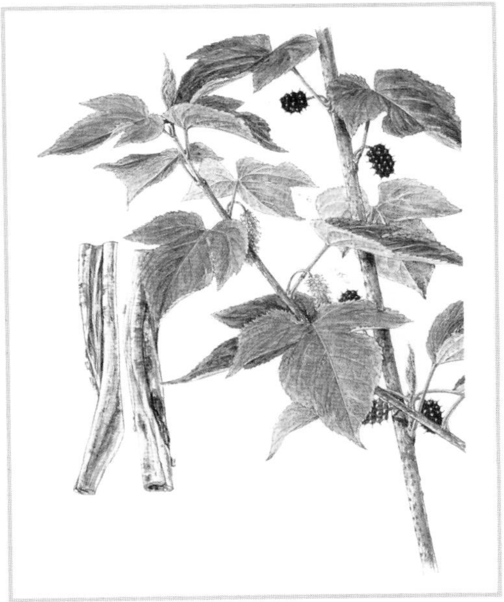

Mori Cortex ▸
[Origin] the cortex of the root of *Morus bombycis* KOIDZ. or other members of the Moraceae family

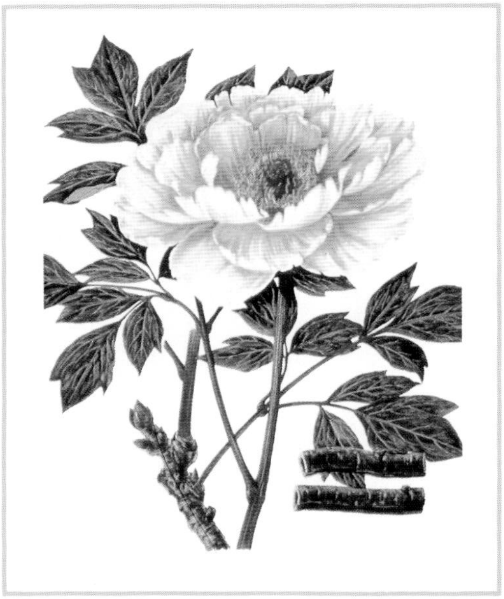

◂ **Moutan Cortex**
[Origin] the cortex of the root of *Paeonia suffruticosa* ANDR. of the Paeoniaceae family

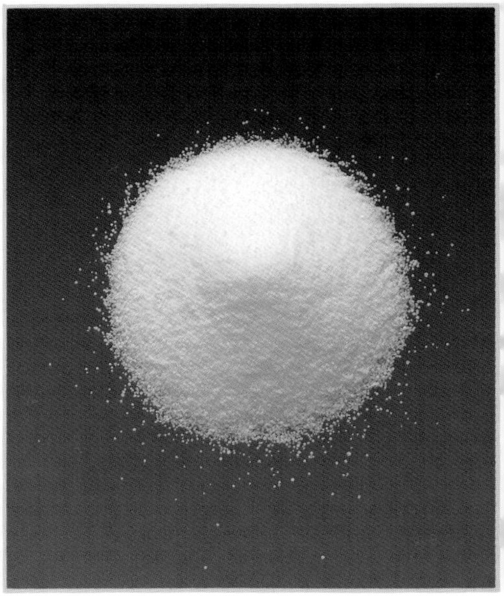

Natrium Sulfuricum ▸
[Origin] natural hydrous sodium sulfate; $Na_2SO_4 \cdot 10H_2O$ or $Na_2SO_4 \cdot 2H_2O$

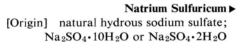

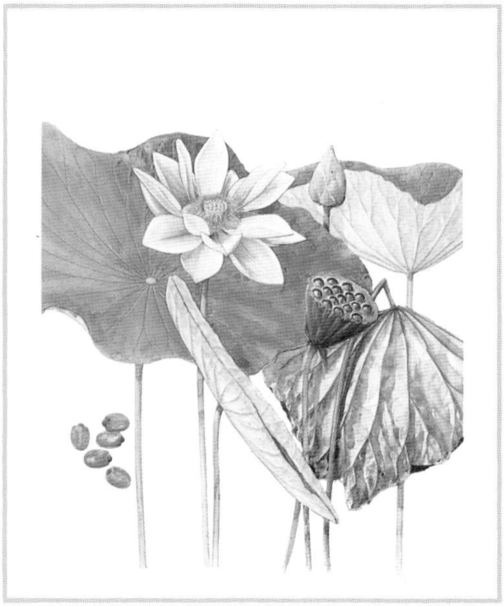

◂ **Nelumbinis Semen**
[Origin] the seed of *Nelumbo nucifera* GAERTN. of the Nymphaeaceae family

Notopterygii Rhizoma ▶
[Origin] the radix and root of *Notopterygium forbesii* BOISS. or other members of the Umbelliferae family

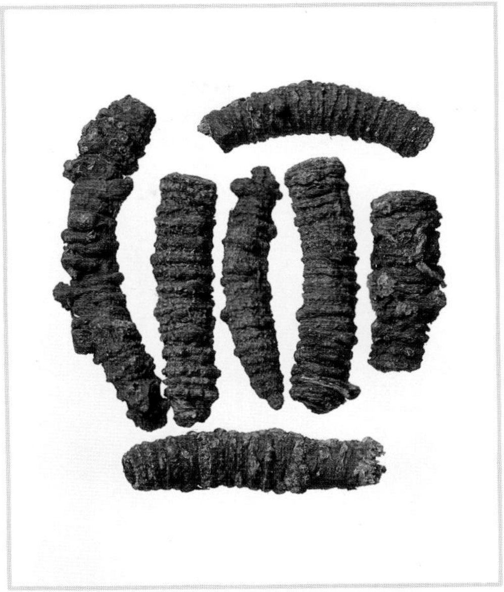

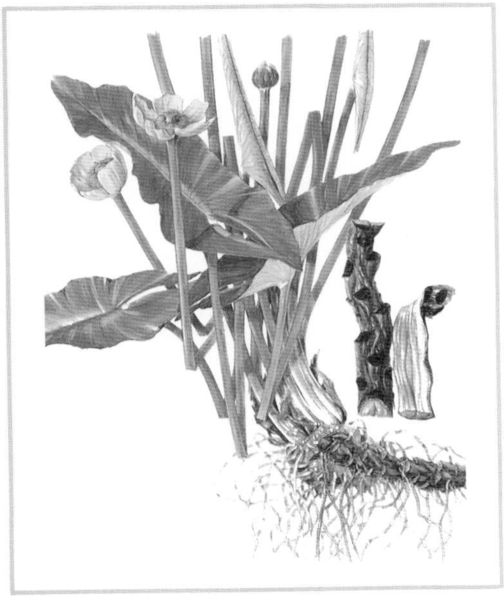

◀ **Nupharis Rhizoma**
[Origin] the longitudinally divided rhizome of *Nuphar japonicum* DC. or other members of the Nymphaeaceae family

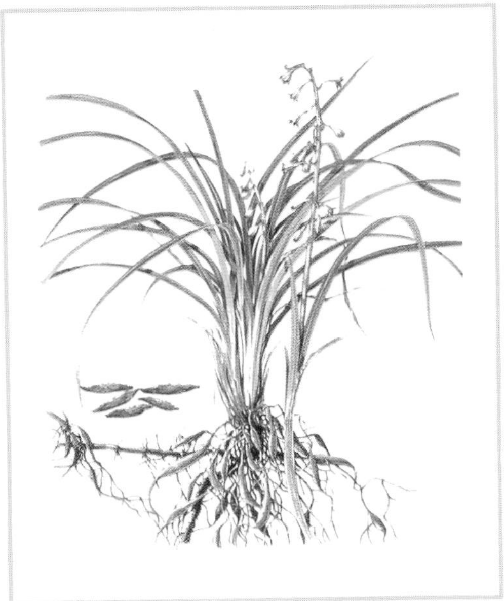

Ophiopogonis Tuber ▶
[Origin] the swollen part of the root of *Ophiopogon japonicus* KER-GAWL. or similar members of the Liliaceae family

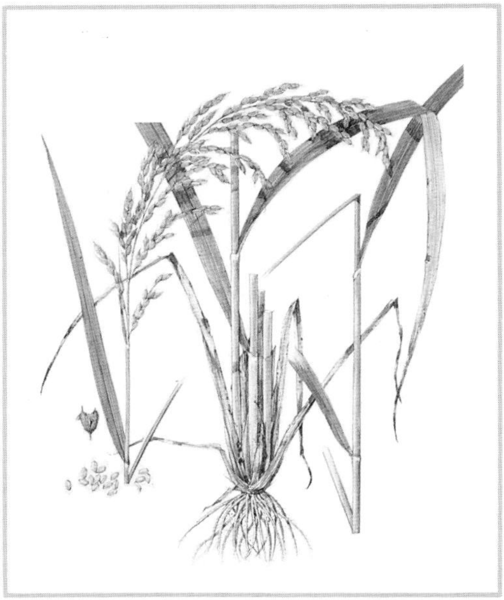

◀ **Oryzae Fructus**
[Origin] the unpolished grain minus chaff of *Oryza sativa* L. of the Gramineae family

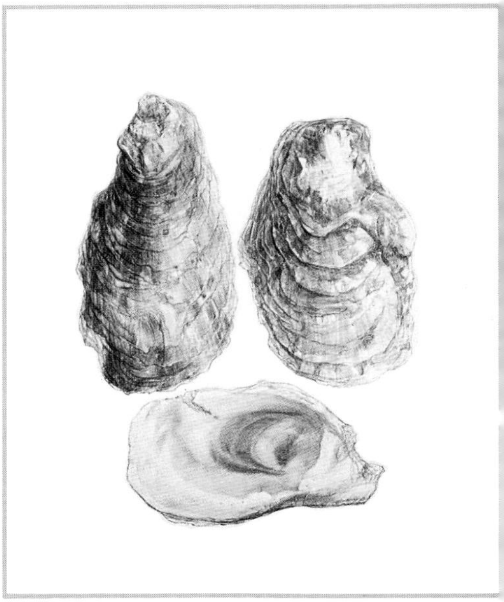

Ostreae Testa ▶
[Origin] the shell of *Ostrea gigas* THUNB. of the Osteridae family

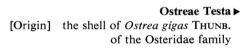

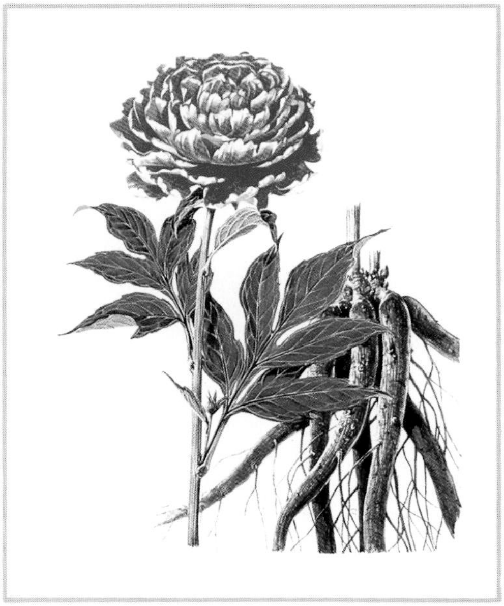

◀ **Paeoniae Radix**
[Origin] the root of *Paeonia lactiflora* PALL. or other similar members of the Paeoniaceae family

Perillae Herba ▶

[Origin] the leaf and the tip of the branch of *Perilla frutescens* BRITT. var. acuta KUDO or similar members of the Labiatae family

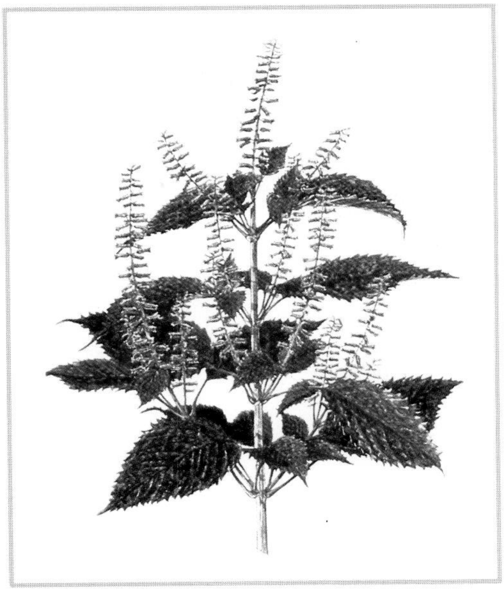

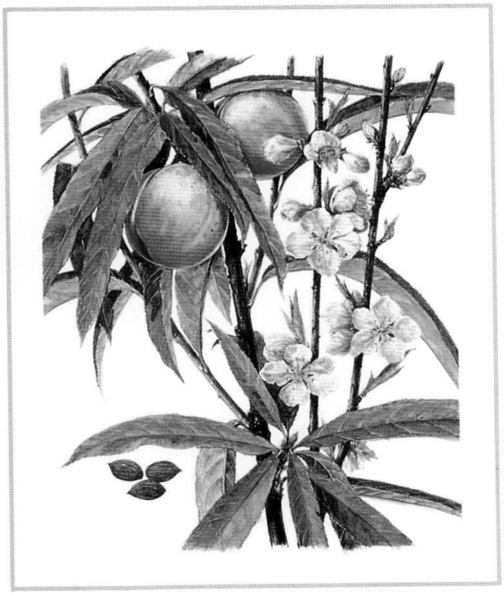

◀ Persicae Semen

[Origin] the seed of *Prunus persica* BATSCH or *P. persica* BATSCH var. *davidiana* MAXIM. of the Rosaceae family

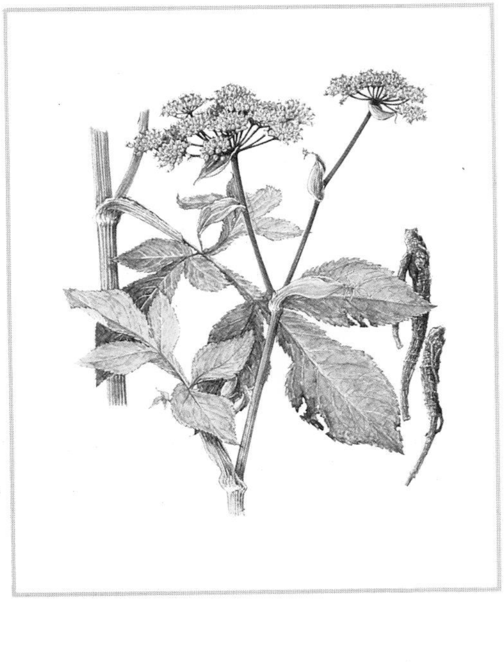

Peucedani Radix ▶

[Origin] the root of *Peucedanum praeruptorum* DUNN. or similar members of the Umbelliferae family

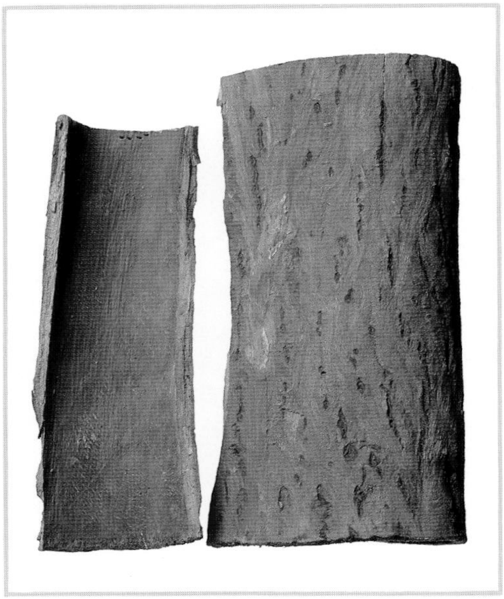

◀ **Phellodendri Cortex**
[Origin] the cortex minus the periderm of *Phellodendron amurense* RUPR. or of other members of the Rutaceae family

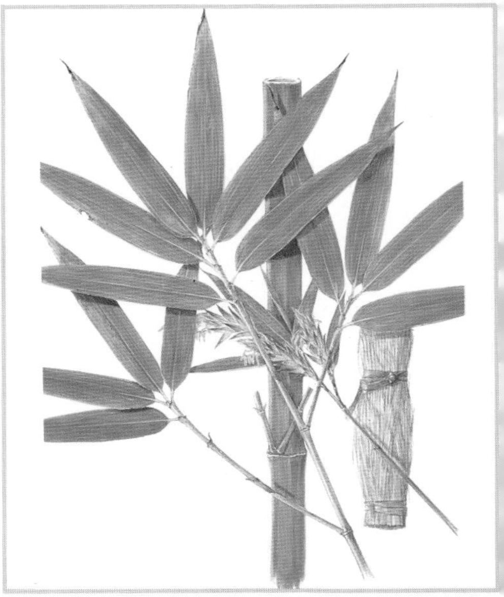

Phyllostachysis Caulis in Taeniam ▶
[Origin] the inside layer after the outside has been removed by scraping of the straw of *Phyllostachys nigra* MUNRO var. *henonis* STAPF ex RENDLE or *P. bambusoides* SIEB. et ZUCC. of the Gramineae family

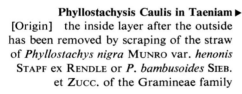

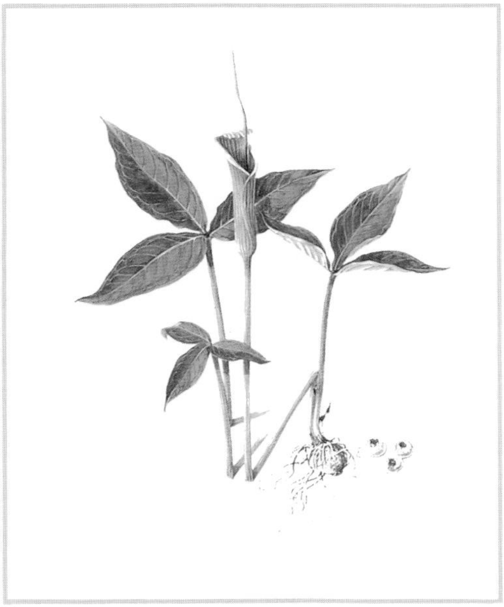

◀ **Pinelliae Tuber**
[Origin] the tuber minus the phelloder of *Pinellia ternata* BREIT. of the Araceae family

Plantaginis Semen ▶
[Origin] the seed of *Plantago asiatica* L. of the Plantaginaceae family

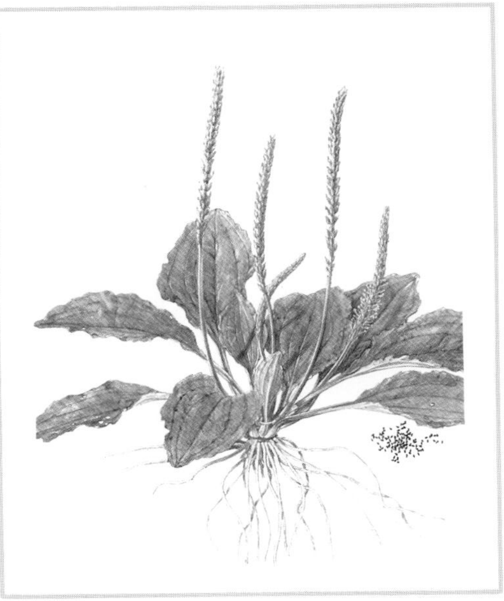

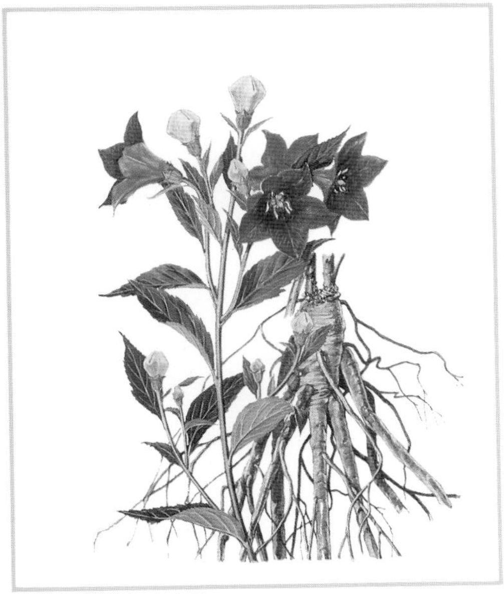

◀ Platycodi Radix
[Origin] the root of *Platycodon grandiflorum* A. DC. of the Campanulaceae family

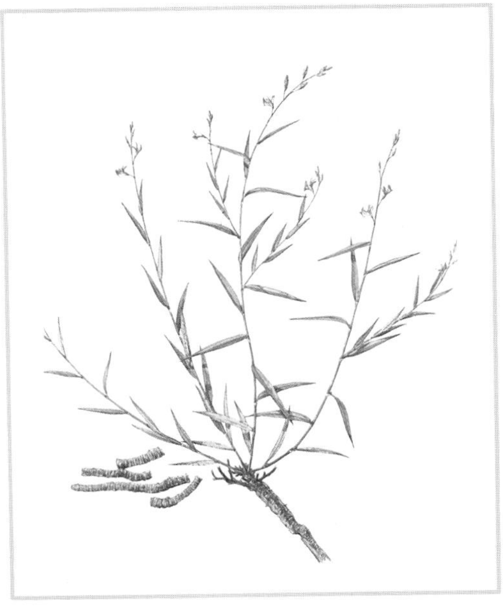

Polygalae Radix ▶
[Origin] the root of *Polygala tenuifolia* WILLD. of the Polygalaceae family

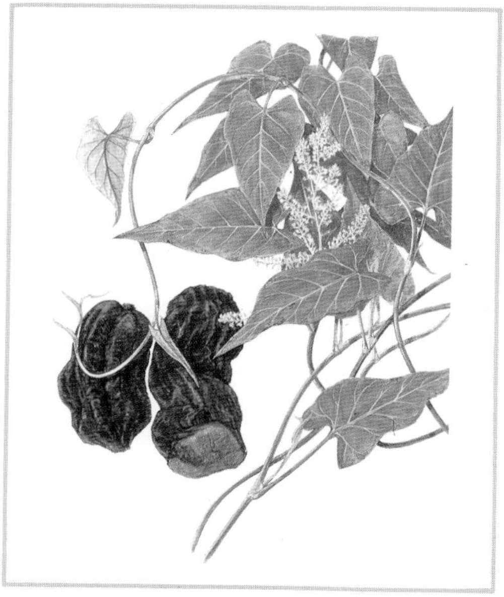

◀ **Polygoni Multiflori Radix**
[Origin] the radix of *Polygonum multiflorum* THUNB. of the Polygonaceae family

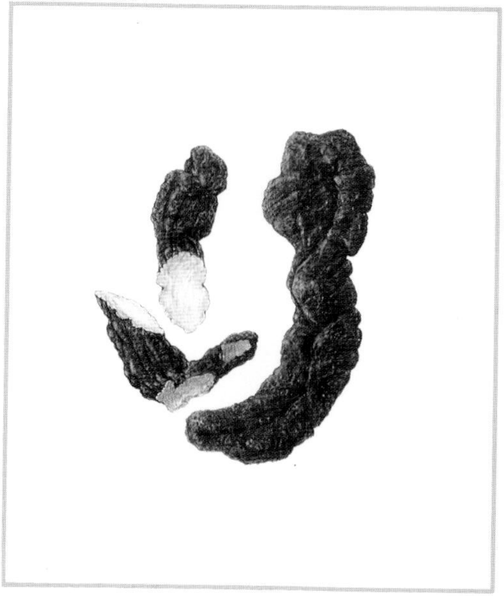

Polyporus ▶
[Origin] the screrotium of *Polyporus umbellatus* FRIES of the Polyporaceae family

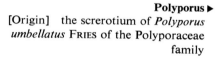

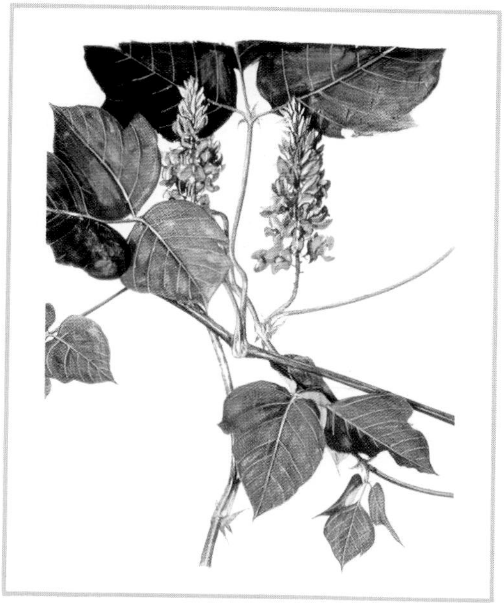

◀ **Puerariae Radix**
[Origin] the root minus the periderm of *Pueraria lobata* OHWI or *P. lobata* OHWI var. *chinensis* (BENTH.) OHWI of the Leguminosae family

Quercus Cortex ▸
[Origin] the cortex of *Quercus acutissima* CARRUTH. or similar members of the Fagaceae family

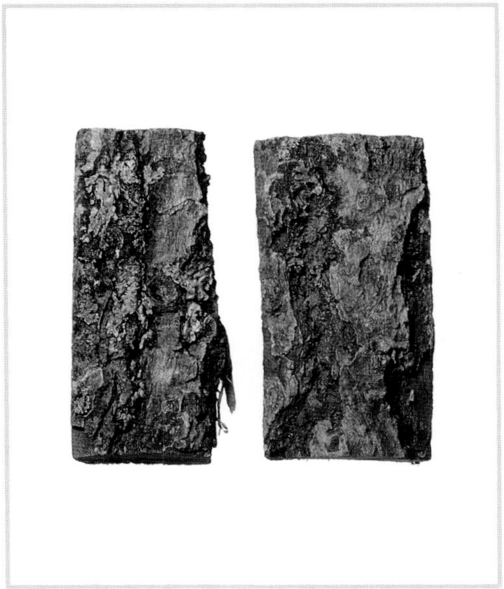

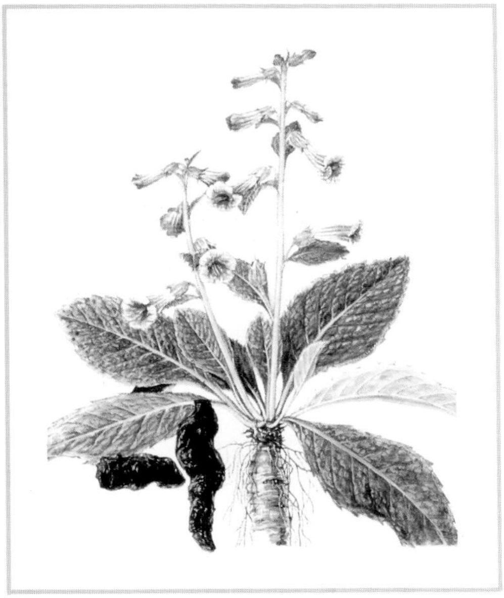

◂ Rehmanniae Radix
[Origin] the dried or steamed whole root of *Rehmannia glutinosa* LIB., var. *purpurea* MAK. or other members of the Scrophulariaceae family

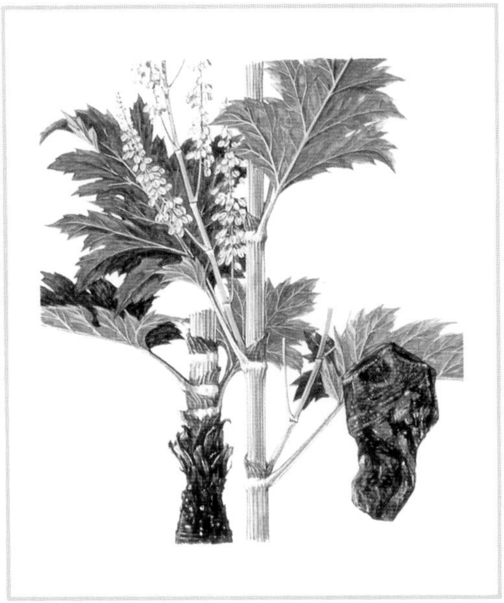

Rhei Rhizoma ▸
[Origin] generally, the rhizome of *Rheum palmatum* L., *R. tanguticum* MAXIM., *R. officinale* BAILL., or the crosses between these species of the Polygonaceae family

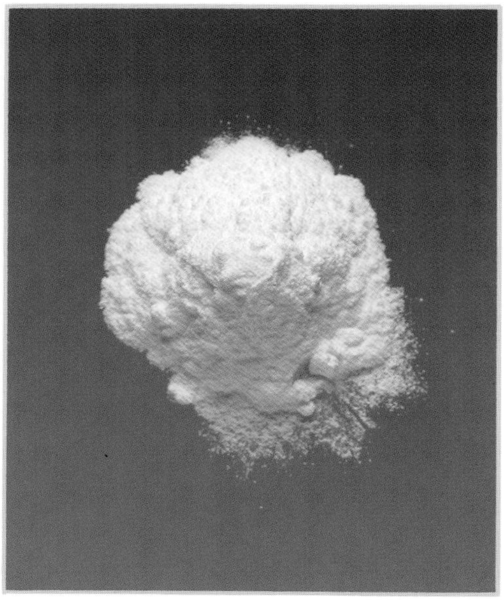

◀ **Saccharum Granorum**
[Origin] candy made from the grain of rice and wheat of the Gramineae family, the grain being powdered, malt added, and saccharified

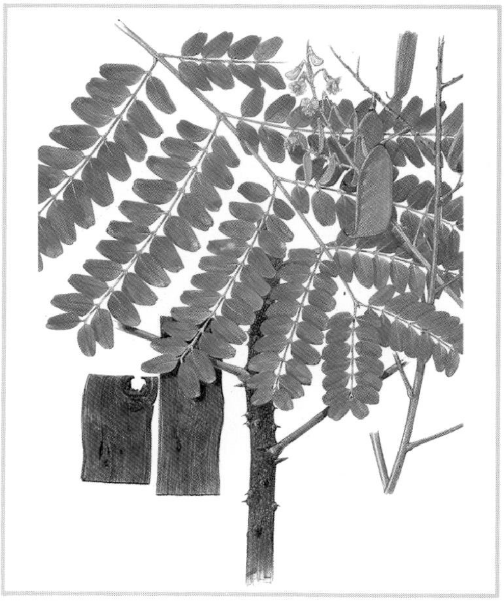

Sappan Lignum ▶
[Origin] the heartwood of *Caesalpinia sappan* L. of the Leguminosae family

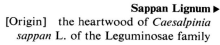

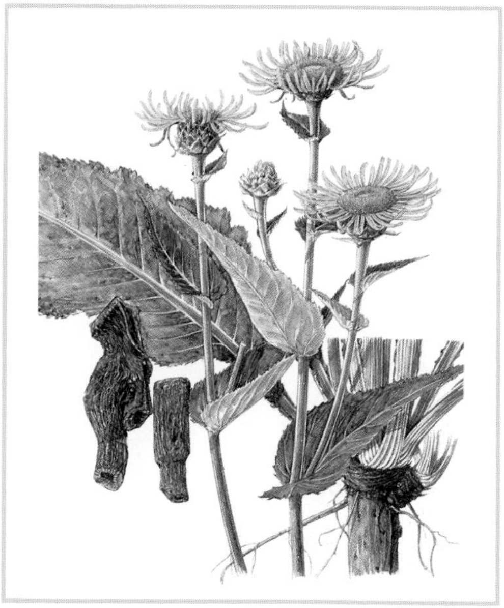

◀ **Saussureae Radix**
[Origin] the root of *Saussurea lappa* CLARKE of the Compositae family

Schisandrae Fructus ▶
[Origin] the fruit of *Schisandra chinensis* BAILL. of the Schisandraceae family

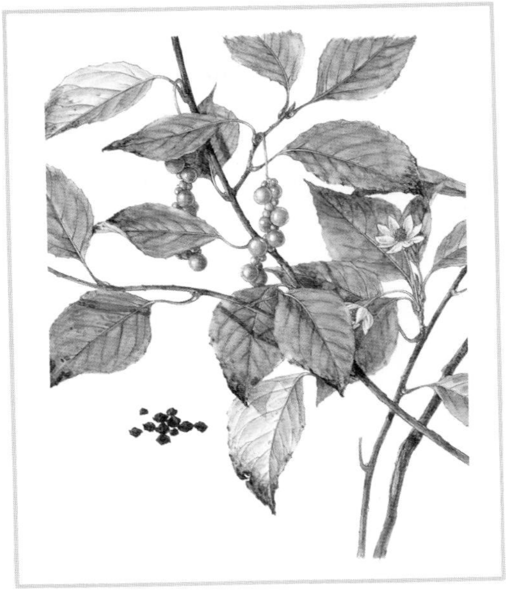

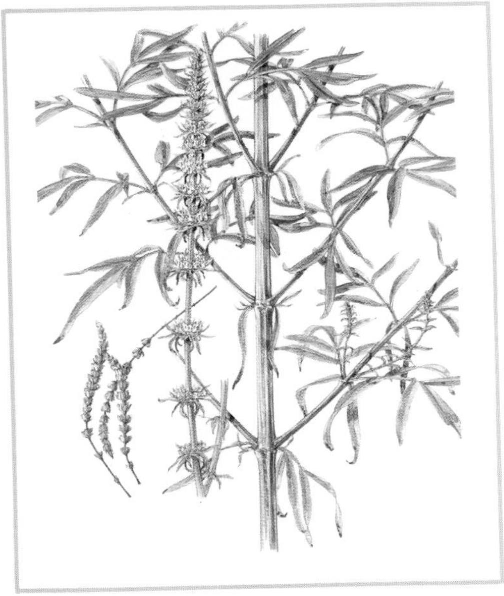

◀ Schizonepetae Spica
[Origin] the head of the flower of *Schnizoepeta tenuifolia* BRIQ. (var. *japonica* KITAGAWA) of the Labiatae family

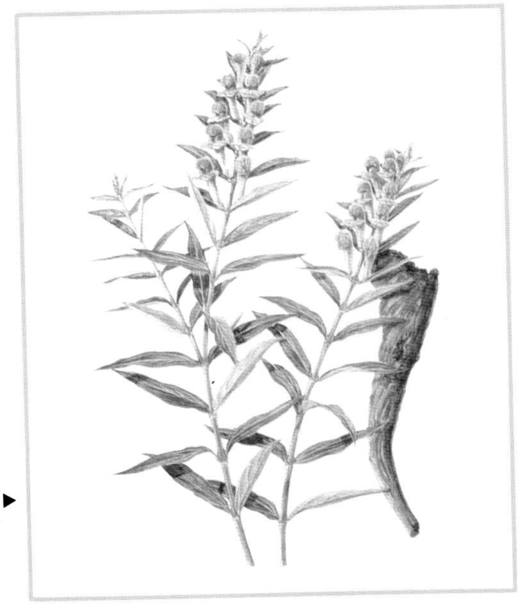

Scutellariae Radix ▶
[Origin] the root minus the periderm of *Scutellaria baicalensis* GEORGI of the Labiatae family

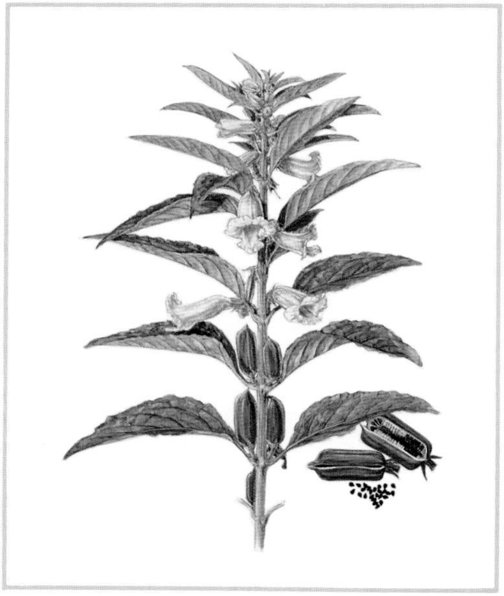

◄ **Sesami Semen**
[Origin] the seed of *Sesamum indicum* L. of the Pedaliaceae family

Sinomeni Caulis et Rhizoma ►
[Origin] the volubile stem or the rhizome of *Sinomenium acutum* REHD. et WILS. of the Menispermaceae family

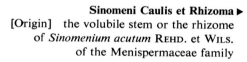

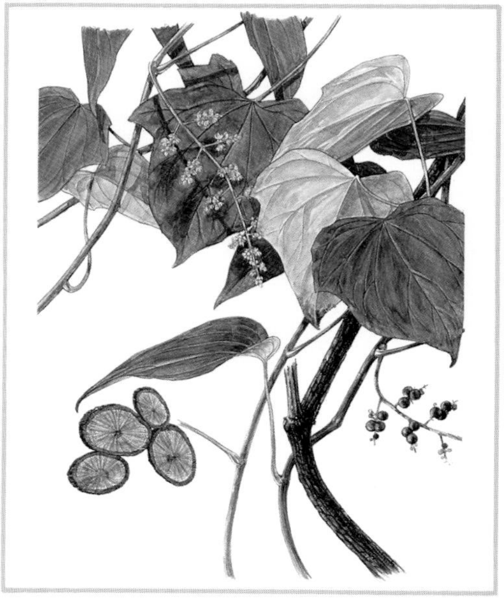

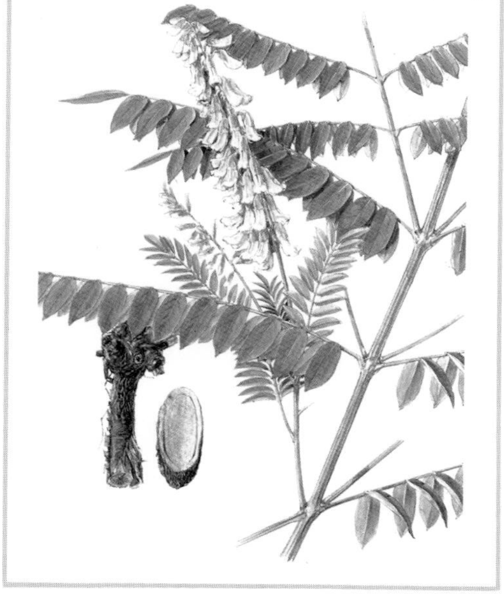

◄ **Sophorae Radix**
[Origin] the root of *Sophora flavescens* AIT. of the Leguminosae family

Swertiae Herba ▸
[Origin] the entire plant of *Swertia japonica* MAKINO of the Gentianaceae family in the flowering season

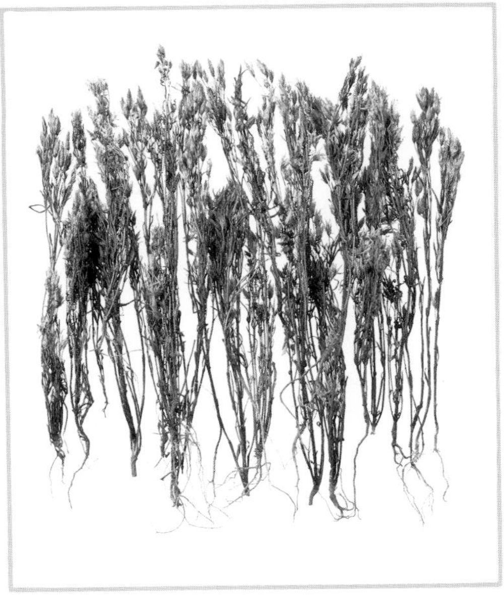

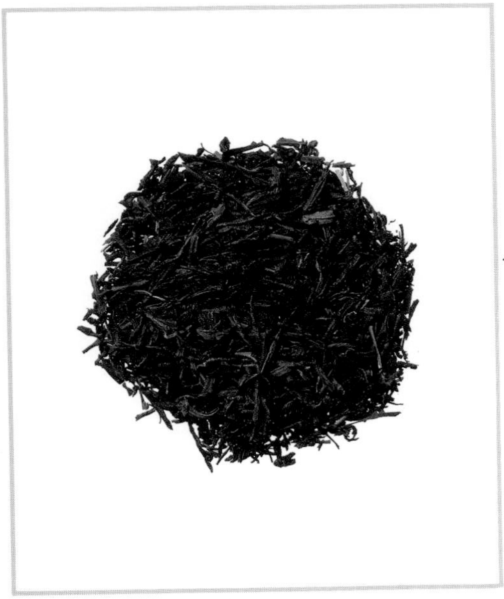

◂ Theae Folium
[Origin] the leaf of *Thea sinesis* L. or other members of the Theaceae family

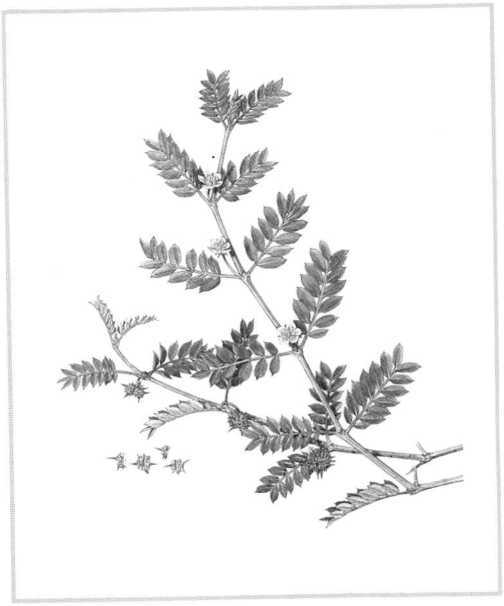

Tribuli Fructus ▸
[Origin] the fruit of *Tribulus terrestris* L. of the Zygophyllaceae family

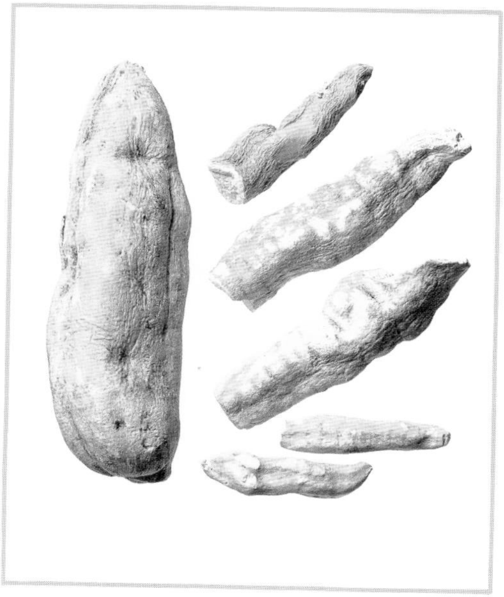

◂ **Trichosanthis Radix**
[Origin] the root minus the cortex of *Trichosanthes kirillowii* MAXIM. var. *japonicum* KITAM., *T. bracteata* VOIGT, or *T. kirillowii* MAXIM. of the Cucurbitaceae family

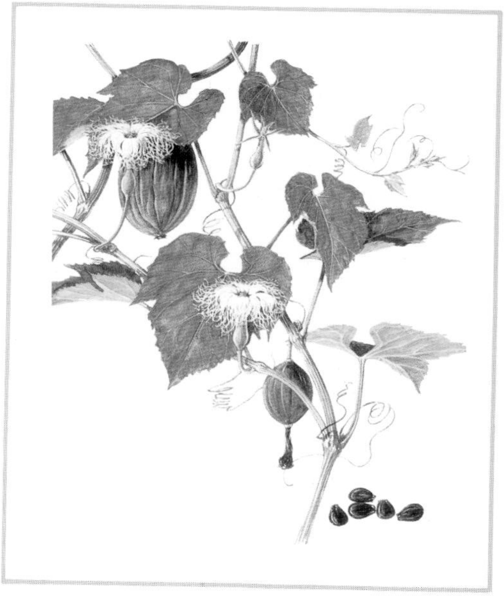

Trichosanthis Semen ▸
[Origin] the seed of *Trichosanthes kirillowii* MAXIM. var. *japonicum* KITAM., *T. bracteata* VOIGT or *T. kirillowii* MAXIM. of the Cucurbitaceae family

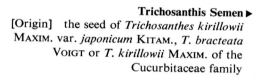

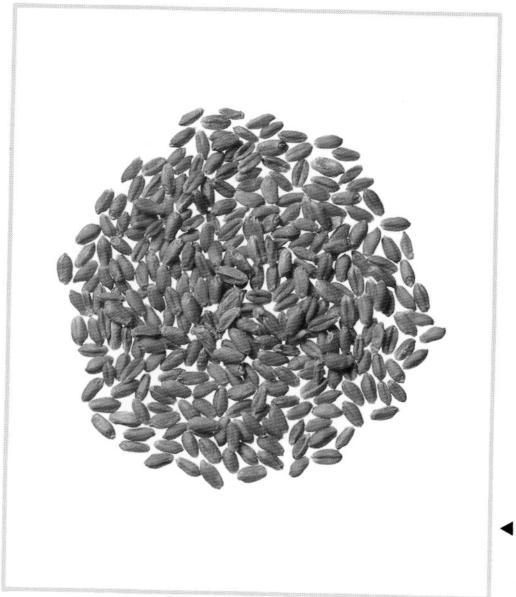

◂ **Tritici Fructus**
[Origin] the seed of *Triticum sativum* LAM. of the Gramineae family

Uncariae Ramulus et Uncus ▶
[Origin] generally, the prickles of *Uncaria rhynchopylla* MIQ. or *U. sinensis* OLIV. of the Rubiaceae family

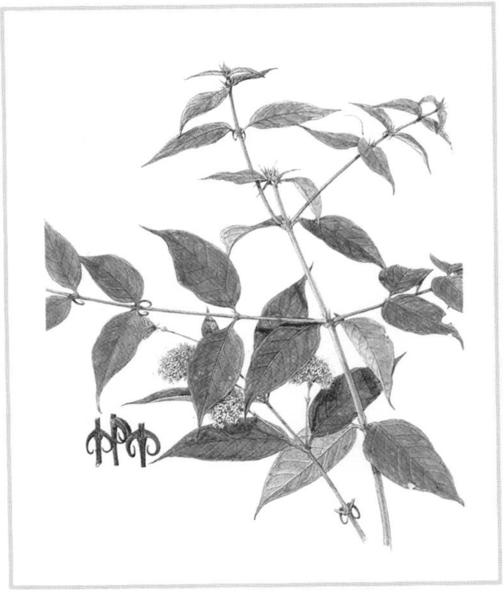

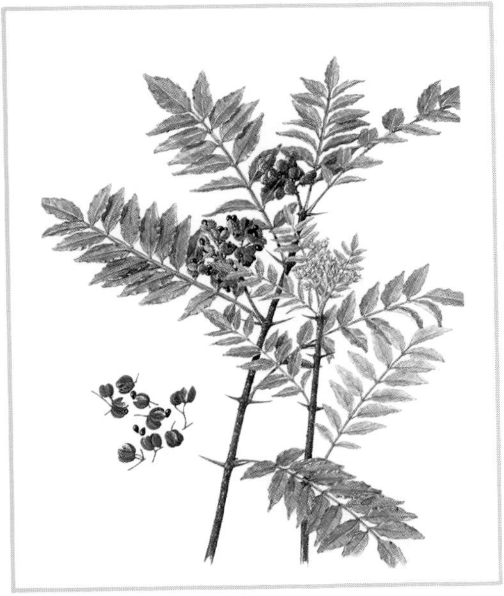

◀ **Zanthoxyli Fructus**
[Origin] the skin of the ripe fruit of *Zanthoxylum piperitum* DC. or other members of the Rutaceae family

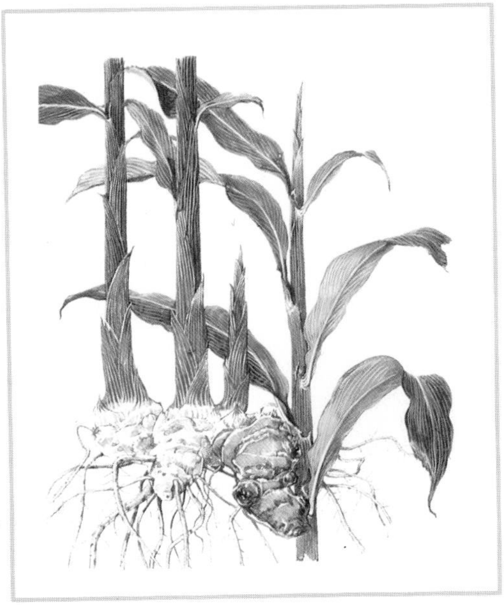

Zingiberis Rhizoma ▶
[Origin] the rhizome of *Zingiber officinale* ROSC. of the Zingiberaceae family

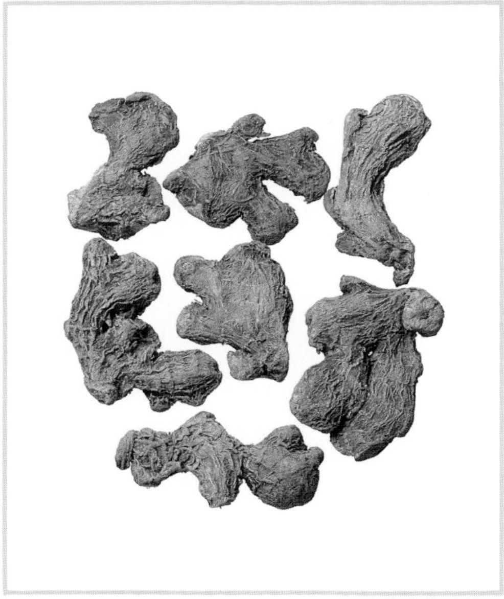

◀ **Zingiberis Siccatum Rhizoma**
[Origin] the rhizome of *Zingiber officinale* Rosc. of the Zingiberaceae family, steamed and phelloderm removed, boiled and dried

Zizyphi Fructus ▶
[Origin] the fruit of *Zizyphus jujuba* MILL. var. *inermis* REHD. or similar members of the Rhamnaceae family

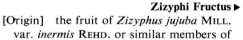

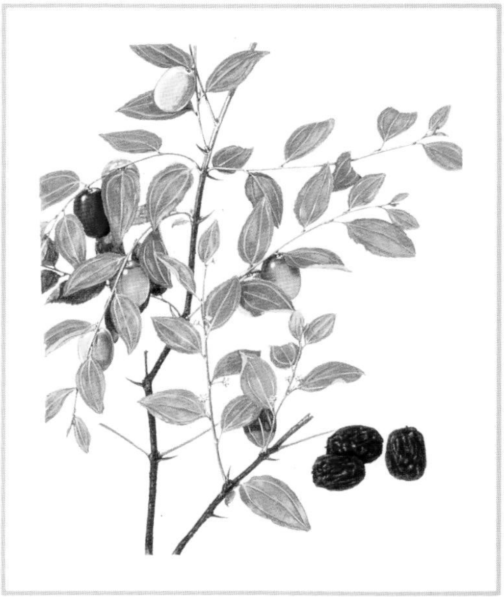

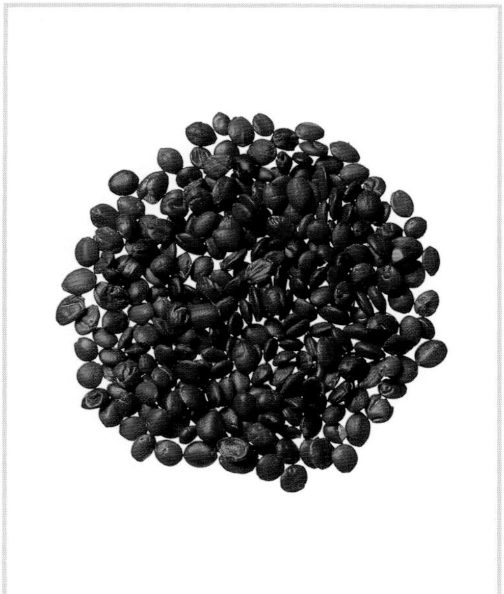

◀ **Zizyphi Spinosi Semen**
[Origin] the seed of *Zizyphus jujuba* MILL. (Z. *vulgaris* LAM. var. *spinosus* BGE.) or other members of the Rhamnaceae family

APPENDICES AND GLOSSARIES

HERBAL NEWSLETTERS

American Herb Association N/I.
P.O. Box 353
Rescue, CA 95672

The Business of Herbs
P.O. Box 559
Madison, VA 22727

Herbalgram
P.O. Box 12602
Austin, TX 78711

Lawrence River of Natural Products
P.O. Box 186
Collegeville, PA 19426

PROFESSIONAL JOURNALS

Economic Botany

Journal of Ethnopharmacology

Journal of Natural Products

Planta Medica

ORGANIZATIONS

American Herb Society
300 Massachusetts Ave.
Boston, MA 02115

SCHOOLS

California School of Herbal Studies
P.O. Box 39
Forestville, CA 95436

Oriental Healing Arts Institute
8820 South Sepulveda Blvd., Suite 205
Los Angeles, CA 90045

East West Master Course in Herbology
(Covers Kampo)
P.O. Box 712
Santa Cruz, CA 95065

SOURCES OF HERBS AND PRODUCTS

CALIFORNIA

Berkeley Health Foods
2311 Shattuck Avenue
Berkeley, CA 94704

Lhasa Karnak Herb Co.
2482 Telegraph Avenue
Berkeley, CA 94704

Steve Mohorko Co.
16803 Ceres Avenue
Fontana, CA 92335

Herbs of Mexico
3859 Whittier Boulevard
Los Angeles, CA 90023

Organic Foods & Gardens
2655 Commerce Way
Los Angeles, CA 90040

Star Herb Company
352 Miller Avenue
Mill Valley, CA 94941

Golden Gate Herbs
P.O. Box 810
Occidental, CA 95465

Nature's Herb Company
281 Ellis Street
San Francisco, CA 94102

The Herb Store
P.O. Box 5756
Sherman Oaks, CA 91403

Taylor's Herb Gardens
1535 Lone Oak Road
Vista, CA 92084

House of Quality Herbs
P.O. Box 14
Woodland Hills, CA 91365

Nature Works
5310 Derry Avenue, Suite H
Agoura, CA 91301

CONNECTICUT

Capriland's Herb Farm
Silver Street
Coventry, CT 06238

Herb's Herbs
P.O. Box 577
New Canaan CT 06840

IDAHO

Lewiston Health Food Center
861 Main
Lewiston, ID 83501

ILLINOIS

Everett Anderson
Route 2
McLeansboro, IL 62859

Kramer's Health Food Store
29 East Adams Street
Chicago, IL 60603

Dr. Michael's Herb Products
5109 North Western Avenue
Chicago, IL 60625

INDIANA

Indiana Botanic Gardens, Inc.
P.O. Box 5
Hammond, IN 46325

Moses J. Troyer—Lone Organic Farm
Route 1, Box 58
Millersburg, IN 46543

MARYLAND

Carroll Gardens
P.O. Box 310
Westminster, MD 21157

MASSACHUSETTS

Blackthorn Gardens
48 Quincy Street
Holbrook, MA 02343

MICHIGAN

International Growers Exchange
Box 397
Farmington, MI 48024

Woodland Herb Farm
Route 1, Box 105
Northport, MI 49670

Harvest Health
1944 Eastern Avenue, SE
Grand Rapids, MI 49507

MISSOURI

Clearwater Farms
Des Arc, MO 63636
(Ginseng Seed)
Geological Botany Company
622 West 67th Street
Kansas City, MO 64113
The Herb Company
206 West Maple
Independence, MO 64050

NEW JERSEY

Meer Corporation
9500 Railroad Avenue
North Bergen, NJ 07047
Le Jardin du Gourmet
Box 245
Ramsey, NJ 07446
Rocky Hollow Herb Farm
Lake Wallkill Road
Sussex, NJ 07461
Well Sweep Herb Farm
317 Mt. Bethel Road
Port Murray, NJ 07865

NEW YORK

Aphrodisia
282 Bleecker Street
New York, NY 10014
Glie Farms
1600 Bathgate Avenue, Bronx
New York, NY 10457
Meadowsweet Herbal Apothecary
77 East 4th Street
New York, NY 10003
Kalustyan Orient Export Trading Co.
123 Lexington Avenue
New York, NY 10010
H. Roth & Son
1577 First Avenue
New York, NY 10028

OREGON

Nichols Garden Nursery
1190 North Pacific Highway
Albany, OR 97321
The Fishers
Route 2, Box 205
Monmouth, OR 97862

PENNSYLVANIA

Andrew Gallant
Route 2
Albion, PA 16401
Tatra Herb Company
222 Grove Street
Morrisville, PA 19067
Haussman's Pharmacy
6th & Girard Avenue
Philadelphia, PA 19127
Penn Herb Company
603 North 2nd Street
Philadelphia, PA 19123
Edward's Health Center
480 Station Road
Quackerstown, PA 18951

RHODE ISLAND

Greene Herb Gardens
Greene, RI 02827
Meadowbrook Herb Garden
Route 138
Wyoming, RI 02898

TENNESSEE

Blue Ridge Ginseng
McDonald, TN 37353

TEXAS

Blue Stage Herb Farm
406 Post Oak Road
Fredericksburg, TX 78624
Plimmers Enterprises
P.O. Box 701
Alpine, TX 79830

VERMONT

Vermont Country Store
Weston, VT 05161

WASHINGTON

Cedarbrook Herb Farm
Route 1, Box 1047
Sequim, WA 98382

WISCONSIN

N'Western Processing Company
217 North Broadway
Milwaukee, WI 53202

CANADA

Botanical Herbs& Health Products
P.O. Box 88 Station "N"
Montreal, Quebec, Canada

Rolly's Health Food Store
634 Yonge Street
Toronto, Ontario, Canada

World-Wide Herb Limited
11 St. Catherine Street E.
Montreal, 129, Quebec, Canada

For Your Health
Box 307
1136 Eglinton Avenue, W.
Willowdale, Ontario, Canada

MEDICAL GLOSSARY

ACUPUNCTURE ə′·kyo͞o·pungk·chər	Insertion of needles into the body at specific areas to work through the autonomic nervous system.
ANTICOAGULANT an′·tī·kō·ag′·y·o͞olənt	Substance that prevents blood clots.
ANTIEMETIC an′·ti·ē·met·ik	Reduces feelings of nausea.
ANTIHISTAMINE an′·tī·his′·tə·mēn	Relieves allergic symptoms.
ANTIMICROBIAL an′·tī·mi·krō′·bē·əl	They help the body resist pathogenic microorganisms, aiding the natural immune processes. "Antibiotics" often do as much harm as good.
ANTITUSSIVE an′·ti·tus′·iv	Remedy to relieve cough.
AORTA ā·ôr′·tə	Largest blood vessel in the body.
ARTERIOSCLEROSIS är·tē″·ri·ō·sklə·rō′·səs	Thickening and loss of elasticity in the arterial walls.
ASTHMA az′·mə	Wheezing, cough, difficulty breathing.
CAPSULE kap′·səl	Soluble, gelatinous container used for a dose of medicine.
CHOLAGOGOUS kelä′geges	Affecting flow of bile.
DIURETIC dī′·yo͞o·ret·ik	An agent that increases the flow of urine.
HEMATOMA hē·mə·tō′·mə	A swelling that contains blood, normally clotted, in an organ, space, or tissue.
HEPATOMA hep·ə·tō′·mə	Tumor of the liver.
HOMEOSTASIS hō·mē·ō·stā′·səs	Physiological equilibrium.
HYPOGLYCEMIA hī·pō·glī·sē′·mē·ə	Condition marked by low blood sugar.
HYPOTENSIVE hī·pō·ten′·siv	Marked by low blood pressure.
INTERFERON in·tər·fēr″·än	Protein substance in body effective against viruses.
MOXIBUSTION moks′i·bus·chən	Counter-irritation by means of a moxa. (Combustible material placed on an acupuncture needle.)
MUCILAGE myoo′·sə·lij	In pharmacology, a thick, viscuous liquid; a water solution of the mucilagenous principles of certain vegetable substances.
NEUROSIS no͞o·rō′·səs	Emotional maladjustments.
OVER-THE-COUNTER ō·vər t͟hə koun′·tər	Medication not requiring a prescription to order.
PALPATE pal′·pāt	Examine patient by touch of the hand as a diagnostic aid.
PATHOGEN path′·ə·jən	Microorganisms causing disease.

PEPSIN pep′·sin	Enzyme in gastric juice that helps digest proteins.
SEDATIVE sed′·ət·iv	Agent that slows down nervous activity.
STIMULANT stim′·yə·lənt	Physicians using strong stimulants must often prescribe potent chemicals to balance overactivity. This is not so in herbalism. Herbal stimulants can all be used safely.
SYNERGY sin′·ər·jē	The quality of two substances when combined to achieve cures beyond their individual effects.

PREFIXES:

hermato	blood
cardio	heart
myo	muscle
ouro	shoulder
osteo	bone
neuro	nerve
arterio	arteries
colo	colon
append	appendix
dent	teeth
oculo	eye
aden	gland
brachi	arm
nephro	kidney
cephal	head
derma	skin
entero	intestine
gastro	stomach
glosso	tongue
hepa	liver
pneu	lungs

SUFFIXES:

algia	pain
oma	tumor
iasis	condition
osis	disease
aclerosis	hardness
cele	cyst
gram	a record
plegia	stroke
phobia	fear
logy	study of
pathy	disease
cyte	cell
itis	inflammation
ectomy	cutting out
trophic	nourishment

Pronunciation Key

a	add, mat, cat	i	liquid, sit, it	ou	out, mouth, snout
ā	fade, weight, mate	ī	blind, right, kind	u	puppet, mud, flutter
â	pair, care, air	o	nostril, mop, top	ng	angry, song, ring
ä	dart, mark, arm	ō	float, hold, told	th	thick, thumb, thought
e	left, web, fed	ô	born, swarm, warn	th̲	the, feather, mother
ə	level, seven, even	oi	moist, boy, toy	hw	what, which, whale
ē	see, bee, meet	oo	look, wood, stood	zh	measure, treasure, azure
ur	fern, turn, worm	o͞o	move, do, fool		

CHEMICAL GLOSSARY

ALKALOIDS ɑl′·kə·loids	Compounds containing a nitrogen atom. Alkaloids are usually present in plants as groups of chemicals. Physical effects include killing pain, poisoning, and causing hallucinations.
ANTHRAQUINONES ɑn′·thrə·kwin·ōns′	Glycoside compounds used in purgatives.
BITTERS bit′·ərs	Herbs containing a wide range of chemicals that have bitter taste. Useful as appetite stimulants, anti-inflammatories, and as relaxants.
CARBOHYDRATES kär′·bō·hī″·drāts	The most common are the nutritionally important sugars and starches, and cellulose. Polysaccharides are sugars that join with other chemicals to produce compounds such as pectin and mucilage which soothe, protect, and relax the alimentary canal.
COUMARINS ko͞o′·mə·rəns	Glycoside compounds that are responsible for the "new mown hay" smell of many grasses.
FLAVONOID GLYCOSIDES flā′·və·noid glī·kə·sīds′	Group of plant chemicals with a wide variety of actions. Used as diuretics, circulatory stimulants, and antispasmodics.
GLYCOSIDES glī·kə·sīds′	Common plant chemicals with a strong effect on the heart (e.g. foxglove/digitalis). Some are purgative (e.g. the anthraquinones in cascara, senna, rhubarb, and buckthorn).
MUCILAGES myo͞o′·sə·lij·əs	Gel-like substances. Soothing effect when applied to inflammed tissues by mimicking the body's own protective mechanism of mucus production.
PHENOL fē′·nōl	Basic building block of many plant constituents such as salicylic acid, often combined with a sugar to form an antiseptic (e.g. in meadowsweet).
SALICYLATES sə·lis″·ə·lāts′	Natural aspirin-type chemicals. They work well, without any danger to the stomach. Aspirin can damage the stomach.
SAPONINS sɑp′·ə·nəns	Glycosides that form a soap-like lather when shaken in water. Two groups: Steroidal saponins which mimic the precursors of female hormones, and the tri-terpenoid saponins, which mimic the adrenal hormone ACTH.
TANNINS tɑn′·əns	Compounds that react with protein to produce a leatherlike coating on animal tissue. They promote healing and numb to reduce irritation. They also reduce inflammation and halt infection.
VOLATILE OILS väl′·ə·tīl oils	These complex compounds are chemical mixtures of hydrocarbons and alcohols. In plants they enhance the moisture-retaining properties of the leaves. They give herbs their characteristic taste and flavor. They are often antiseptic, antifungal, and aromatic. Volatile oils also enhance digestion, prevent flatulence, and calm the nervous system.

PLANT GLOSSARY

ACHENE ə·kēn′	A small, dry fruit that contains one loose seed and that does not split open spontaneously (e.g., sunflower seed).
BLADE blād	The broad, thin part of a leaf or petal.
BLOOM blo͞om	A powdery, whitish coating on plants.
BRACT brakt	Small, sometimes scale-like leaf, usually associated with flower clusters.
BULB bulb	A thick, rounded underground organ consisting of layered, fleshy leaves and membranes.
CORM kôrm	A bulblike but solid, fleshy underground stem base.
COROLLA kə·räl′·ə	The petals of a flower.
CREEPER krē′·pər	A shoot that grows along the gound, rooting all along its length.
CULM kəlm	The hollow stem of grasses and bamboos.
DRUPE dro͞op	A fleshy fruit containing a single seed in a hard "stone" (e.g., peach).
FLORET flor′·ət	Small flower in a flower head or cluster.
FROND frond	The leaf of a fern.
FRUIT fro͞ot	The seed bearing part of a plant.
HESPERIDIUM hes′·pə·rid″·ē·əm	A partitioned berry with a leathery, removable rind (e.g., orange).
LEGUME leg′·yo͞om	A one-celled fruit that splits along two seams (e.g., pea).
NODE nōd	Place where a leaf grows or can grow.
NUT nut	A hard-walled, one-seeded fruit that does not split spontaneously (e.g., hazelnut).
PEDICEL ped′·ə·səl	The stalk of one flower in a cluster.
PISTIL pist′·əl	Female reproductive organ of a flower.
POD pod	Generally, a dry fruit that splits open.
POME pōm	Fleshy fruit with a central seed-bearing core (e.g., apple).
PROCUMBENT prō·kəm′·bənt	Growing along the ground without rooting, and having ascending tips.
RADICAL rod′·i·kəl	Growing from or pertaining to a root; growing from a non-aerial stem.
RECEPTACLE ri·sep′·ti·kəl	The end of the stem or stalk on which the flower parts are borne.

RHIZOME rī′·zōm	Underground portion of a stem, producing shoots on top and roots beneath; different from a root in that it has buds, nodes, and scaly leaves; rootstock.
RUNNER run′·ər	Thin stem or shoot growing along the ground and producing roots at the nodes.
SCOPE skōp	Leafless flower stalk growing along the ground.
SHRUB shrub	Woody plant with no trunk but branches growing from base.
SPORE spôr	One-celled reproductive body produced by primitive plants.
STAMEN stā·mən	The male or pollen-bearing organ of a flower.
STYLE stīl	Slender, elongated part of a pistil.
TAPROOT tap′·rōōt″	A single, main root growing vertically into the ground.
TUBER tōō′·bər	A thick, fleshy part, usually of a rootstock.

BIBLIOGRAPHY

Baker, H.G., *Plants and Civilization*, Wadsworth Publishing, Belmont, CA, 1966

A Barefoot Doctor's Manual (Oriental Therapies) Chicago: Cloudburst Press, 1977

David Hoffman, *The Herbal Handbook*, Rochester, VT: Healing Arts Press, 1985

Huxley, Anthony, *Green Inheritance*, New York: Anchor Press, Doubleday, 1986

Kloss, Jethro, *Back to Eden*, Riverside, CA: Lifeline Books, 1985

Lust, John, *The Herb Book*, New York: Bantam Books, 1974

Mabey, Richard, *New Age Herbalist*, New York: Collier Books, Macmillan, 1988

Reid, Daniel, *Chinese Herbal Medicine*, Boston: Shambhala Press, 1987

Tierra, Michael, *The Way of Herbs*, New York: Pocket Books, 1980

Treben, Maria, *Health from God's Garden*, Rochester, VT: Thorson's Publishers, 1987

Tyler, Brady, and Robbers, *Pharmacognosy*, New York: Lea and Febigler, 1977

Index of Kampo Medications

General Index

Index of Botanical Names

[illegible]
惟王叔和能學之。其間如葛洪陶景胡洽徐之才
孫思邈輩。非不才也。但各自名家。而不能脩明之。
開寶中。節度使高繼沖。曾編錄進上。其文理舛錯。
未嘗考正。歷代雖藏之書府。亦闕於讎校。是使治
病之流。舉天下無或知者。國家詔儒臣。校正醫書。
臣奇續被其選。以為百病之急。無急於傷寒。今先
校定張仲景傷寒論十卷。總二十二篇。證外合三
百九十七法。除複重。定有一百一十二方。今請頒
行。太子右贊善大夫臣高保衡。尚書屯田員外郎